# On the Sneak Tip: The Male Pelvis Revealed

Written by

Becca Ironside

ISBN: 9798636314271 (paperback)

*For Henry, who wore the boot on the cover of this book;
Despite great hardship, he strode through the world with
grace and tenacity*

# Prologue

In 2006, I accepted a job working as a physical therapist for the city of Newark, NJ. Many of my patients were police officers who sustained injuries on the job as they leapt over fences and ran after criminals on foot, got into motor vehicle accidents during high speed chases or simply developed carpal tunnel syndrome from typing too many reports at a desk. These police officers wore leather belts which weighed over 25 pounds. The cops who came into this physical therapy clinic were responsible for the location and safety of their own guns. The city was supposed to provide gun lockers for the officers, yet as the city of Newark has never been known for having a cushy budget from which to draw, the cops hooked their gun belts onto the arms of coat racks, rested them on chairs, or slid them under treatment tables amongst tubs of massage cream and rolls of athletic tape while they were getting stretched or performed exercises. In short, there were unsecured weapons everywhere, at any given time of day. Upon imagining this scenario, one might think the workers of the clinic would feel unsafe in this environment; but we never did. Instead, we felt safe in the knowledge that we were surrounded by people who had strong knowledge and practice in how to wield firearms.

I learned a lot about men in working with the police force at that time. The force was predominantly male, and they behaved with the bravado, confidence and law enforcement intuition that makes for great cops. They also confided in me, as I was a neutral person in the thick of the battle within their jobs. I had never met many of the higher-ups or that Captain who nobody wanted to work under. During this same time, an enormous political upset had occurred.

Sharpe James had been elected as the Mayor of Newark since 1986. He was re-elected for a total of five four-year terms thereafter. Sharpe James was beloved by the people of Newark. He was one of their own, and he was witnessed walking through local neighborhoods. When the people of Newark were hosting a BBQ, they invited their own mayor to attend. Sharpe James was the kind of guy who would show up in their backyards, crack open a can of Miller Lite, and spend time with the people of Newark. Mr. James stepped down from his leadership in 2006 when he was convicted on five counts of fraud for rigging the sale of some plots of land to his mistress. Sharpe James served time in federal prison for these indictments. It was at this time when Cory Booker took over as the new mayor in town.

Cory Booker was a very different kind of guy than his predecessor Sharpe James. Cory Booker was an educated man who had been raised in the suburbs and then attended Stanford and Yale University. Mr. Booker put many laws in place to allow the residents of Newark to attain affordable housing and he also began an initiative to decrease crime in the city. It all seemed so perfect, right? In the battle of good versus evil, Sharpe James was behind bars and Cory Booker was the proverbial Robin Hood who stole from the rich to save the poor.

Only it wasn't all that simple. Mr. Booker's initiative to decrease crime was successful for a short while. He did expand the police presence throughout town, the accessibility of affordable housing quadrupled for the residents and the city's financial deficit was slashed in half. Yet as time wore on, it became clear that Cory Booker was just another politician. When he was gifted the sum of $100 million to address the dismal school systems of Newark by Facebook's Mark Zuckerberg in 2010, the people of Newark were not surprised to discover that very little would change for the education of their children. So, where did all that money go? It also did not help that Cory Booker was not accessible to the people in his city. Unlike Sharpe James, Cory Booker would not go to those backyard BBQ's and drink Miller Lite. He didn't exude trustworthiness. And the cops? Let's just say that their opinion Cory Booker was unflattering, and they recalled the good old days under Sharpe James with wistful grins.

As this political embroilment was just beginning to unfurl in 2006, I learned an important turn of phrase from the cops of Newark. The definition of the expression "on the sneak tip" is difficult to find on the Internet, though people who know the term understand it to mean *something which is confided in secret, something on the down low, or information imparted covertly which is not to be openly disclosed.* When one of the police officers was divulging something to me, he often prefaced the intel as being "on the sneak tip." I grew to love the phrase, and I also liked being the Keeper of the Deep Well of Secrets for my patients. I thought I had learned everything about men back then. I had mastered the art of getting into their skulls, and of getting them to speak freely. In short, I had become Sharpe James, someone to confide in, without the criminal past or prison sentence.

I had been completely wrong about that. It wasn't until several years later when I became a pelvic floor physical therapist for men that I really began to understand them. Pelvic floor physical therapy specializes in the muscles of the saddle or undercarriage. This type of physical therapy treats men with conditions like urinary leakage, erectile dysfunction, penile and testicular pain, chronic constipation and prostate cancer. These symptoms can happen to men of all ages, from 18 to 89. Perhaps you have never heard of this specialty; many people haven't. Especially men. They may have been dealing with pelvic floor dysfunction, but they are likely not going to tell anyone or get treatment until the severity of the problem overtakes them. There are more men out there with these problems than the medical establishment can discern, because men are so reluctant to talk about their penises.

This book talks all about such problems. It offers a glimpse into what is happening in the groin, how arousal and ejaculation occur, what makes for better bowel movements, how to get more rigid erections and how to address urinary leakage or dribbling. Another feature of this book is what to do in the wake of a diagnosis of prostate cancer, which is the second most commonly diagnosed cancer in the United States. This book is divided into three segments. The first section begins as a fictional account of four men of very different backgrounds with different pelvic problems and one female doctor who treats erectile dysfunction. The second part of the book is nonfiction. It includes studies on why pelvic floor physical therapy works and what other treatment strategies exist for erectile dysfunction, pelvic pain, urinary leakage and prostate cancer. It's a basic How-To-Guide of overall pelvic health for any man. The third and final part of the book is the backstory of the characters. It describes how their conditions affect their lives and how they represent millions of men who have exactly these problems.

The year of 2006 was my very beginning in the study of how men think and operate. It was based on exposure to men in law enforcement during a very heated time in a gritty, rough and tumble town. Since then, I have been exposed to men who have urinary, sexual and bowel concerns, so the stories I am hearing these days are very different than the ones I heard from the police officers. But that beginning in 2006 was important. The mayoral shift from Sharpe James to Cory Booker was crucial in understanding how men are perceived. One would think that Cory Booker would have been the obvious favorite in terms of leadership. But he wasn't. Perhaps that was because he was not seen as like-minded or interested in being part of the city of Newark. Whereas Sharpe James, with his backroom deals and criminal past, was a guy to whom the citizens could say something "on the sneak tip" and feel understood. Sharpe James was perceived as trustworthy, and that made all the difference.

This is not a book about politics. It is a story of men who are desperate to have one person, any person, to talk to about their problems. I had no vested interest in the political landscape of Newark when I worked there many years ago. Instead, my job was to take care of the police officers who were protecting both me and the city of Newark. What I learned about these cops was that they needed a person to talk to. Mayor Sharpe James was the man who understood how difficult it was for the cops. They were able to reach out to him and get what they needed, with less red tape than they found under the administration of Cory Booker. Men need to talk about things; only they have very few avenues down which to travel and be vulnerable in this world. Our society doesn't allow for male expression of weakness, loss or disappointment.

The information given within this book is a compilation of the stories of many men, all of whom have struggled with pelvic problems and have never spoken about them. It is my hope that you as the reader can envision yourself at a backyard BBQ with an open can of beer (even if you don't like beer or Miller Lite, for that matter), and that these men are entrusting you with their very souls. They are telling you things they have never told anyone before. And they are saying them "on the sneak tip."

# Part I

## The Fiction

# Tom

M eet Tom. He was raised in an upper-class neighborhood in New England. Tom's father Dean was a physicist who had gone to Yale, as had all the men in their family for generations before. Tom's parents had old money, the kind of money that was hidden beneath the clapboard of their summer beach house in Nantucket. There was nothing showy about this type of wealth, nor was there room in Tom's future to live a life that strayed from going to Yale or becoming something other than what his father expected of him. The implicit message of Tom's childhood and adolescence was that he was supposed to become his father and continue the family's legacy of wealth, education and privilege.

Tom had the biggest argument of his life with his father Dean when he decided to get a culinary degree. Dean had not gotten his PhD in physics for his only son to become nothing more than a cook. Tom fought his father, they shouted in a way that shook the floorboards of the 19th century center hall colonial like never before. No one had ever fought this argument against the wealth and status of this family. Tom did not care. Instead, Tom enrolled in the culinary program of Johnson and Wales University in Providence, Rhode Island.

Providence was a small metropolis, one which stood in the shadow of her neighboring city, Boston. Tom took every class of cooking school with diligence. He quickly learned the subtleties of a bearnaise sauce, how to sear a steak to perfection and the art of chopping shallots to salvage any dish from disaster. It was not only his skill in cooking that made Tom certain that his decision was the right one. The wintry air off the bay in Rhode Island froze his nostrils as he strode with purpose towards his classes. It was that sharp, briny air that took Tom away from his past.

Providence spoke words of possibility. This city had the whiff of old fishermen who had no other trade but to yank cod from the frigid waters. Tom took that city and whipped her into his own fantasy. In Rhode Island, Tom was a fair distance from his father's expectations. He rose to the top of his class as a chef. All the failings and insults from his childhood (*Tommy's a faggot! What kind of asshole likes to cook for his whore mother?! I guess Tommy can't fix a car, his Daddy has someone to fix his BMW!*) receded into the distance. Tom developed the essential skills of smelling herbs, tasting cheeses and selecting just the right cut of meat with his fingertips as his guide. Cooking was like sex. All the inadequate groping of teenaged girls in the backseat of his car was replaced by something that every man wanted. Tom now had a way to reel in women, and not just girls, like never before.

Something odd happened, though. While Tom could have bagged any chick on campus, there was this one woman named Casey. She was quiet, studious and had a cutely upturned nose. Casey was enrolled at Johnson and Wales as a pastry chef. When Casey was creating a dessert, she had no time for anyone or anything. Tom saw this intensity within her. It was unbelievably hot. Tom watched Casey through the glass windows of the bakery within the University. There came a day when she finished preparing Baked Alaska and returned his gaze at last.

Tom and Casey had sex two weeks later. It was insane sex. In a good way. And it was not in the back seat of a car, either. Tom had booked a hotel room over the water of the city. They went at it all night. Three years later, they got married.

Now, Tom and Casey have two girls together. Casey no longer works the weekends of a pastry chef. This is because she began her own online specialty dessert business. Tom has moved on from being a chef. Due to his remarkable skill in deciphering smell and taste, Tom has become a sommelier. Many people disparage his craft. They say that tasting wine and pairing it with food is just a bunch of horseshit. "Is that a real job?" They ask him. Tom just smiles and laughs all the way to the bank. After all, he is employed by a premier wine magazine. He flies all over Europe to meet with winemakers and is handsomely paid to do so. But more important than his remuneration is the pride that Tom takes in his work. He can detect the green apple undertones of a New Zealand Sauvignon Blanc or a year of Pinot Noir from California where the rain which came from the south was just a bit to mild to deliver the perfect scent of autumn leaves from the glass before sipping.

Everything was going so well. Until it wasn't. Isn't that the way life works? Tom has been married to his wife for eighteen years. The girls are now preteens. Casey's business is thriving, she has her own brand of online desserts. Tom travels for work and he begins to feel an ache in his pelvis. It starts as a small nag if he sits for too long. Tom experiences constipation when he is overseas. He attributes that to the increased barometric pressure on the plane and to poor dietary habits when he is away.

Tom craves sex with his wife Casey. She is more than ready when his plane lands down. But Tom is feeling increasing pressure and pain in his perineum. It gets worse after having sex. It also stabs at him during the bowel movements he needs when he is finally home. When he is not traveling for work, Tom drives his daughters to school and picks then up afterwards. Their chatter used to be amusing. Now, the pain in his rectum and testicles is so severe that he longs for them to shut up.

"How could this have happened to me?" Tom wonders. He wracks his brain for solutions. He pours wine for himself at two in the morning. Casey does not know about his secretive wine drinking. She also does not know of the searing pain that accompanies having sex with him. This woman is Tom's every-thing. Because of this, he refuses to say a word.

Tom looks through the Internet on his phone to find the number of a good urologist. The sun comes up as Tom realizes he has not slept all evening and that one of his favorite bottles of Sangiovese is empty on the soapstone counter. He brings it out to the recycling bin before Casey wakes up.

# Rick

Nobody would choose to be a plumber. It is not one of those things that a guy aspires to be. When Rick was in kindergarten class and the teacher asked, "Who wants to snake toilets and run water lines through a basement?" Rick never raised his hand. Not that the teacher said those actual words, but Rick would grow to learn what it meant to be a plumber. He was not that smart; or so he thought. Middle and high school did not come easily to him. And Rick's father owned the largest plumbing company in all of Pittsburgh.

Pittsburgh was an underrated city in the 1980's. The steel working business had dried up, and a recession had settled on the town. The gloomy weather did not help with the pessimistic outlook on the financial recovery of Pittsburgh. But if you were born there, if your great-grandfather had been a coal miner from Allegheny County and you lived in the same house your father had been born in, it was the best place to live in America.

Rick loved Pittsburgh. He was a Steelers fan to his core. He had played football in high school in Moon Township. He was not the best running back, but he was reliable when he threw the ball. Rick's parents sat on the stone-cold seats of the high school bleachers; they had watched every single game. His mother cooked him a pound of bacon afterwards. His father, Dick, sat on an old recliner in the living room, reading *The*

*Pittsburgh Post-Gazette*, as he watched John Wayne movies. Although Dick was not at the kitchen table eating that pound of bacon with his teenaged boy after those victorious games, the pride for his son bled throughout the house.

Rick had a good life from childhood, through his teenaged years and even as an adult. When he decided not to go to college, Rick's father gave him an apprenticeship in the plumbing business. It was hard work. There was heavy manual labor, one had to unclog sewer lines in old basements, tear out old galvanized pipes and replace them copper. Nobody wanted to pay for copper. Especially in the poorer sections of town. But Rick had the gift of gab, and he talked these people into better pipes, plumbing that would last in these old, brick homes. Everyone trusted Rick. He was not the kind of guy to screw anyone over, especially those who had known his grandfather. He often gave discounts to customers down on their luck, and he fixed the books so that his father Dick never figured it out.

Rick got married to the bookkeeper of the business, Nicole. She had started working there when Rick was 24. It was never hot and heavy, so to speak, but they a good camaraderie. Rick took Nicole to the hot spots in Shadyside, but she was not the kind of girl that needed swank dinners out. They had a simple companionship, and Nicole's mother was ill and longed for her daughter to marry. They planned a wedding at a community center on Neville Island. Rick rented a tuxedo and all his high school friends attended the event.

Rick's father retired and left the business to his son and his wife. Rick and Nicole took over *Dick and Son Plumbing* and life was sweet and good. They bought a house and Nicole got pregnant with their first child. Despite the hard-luck image of Pittsburgh, this business made real money. It cleared over $80,000 annually. (This was like making $160,000 in Connecticut. And this was in the 1990's!)

Rick and Nicole had only one son, named Francis, after Rick's grandfather. Thereafter, Nicole suffered multiple miscarriages. She wept through the night as Rick held her close. They attempted infertility treatments, but Nicole finally put her foot down. She was too depressed to continue down a journey that she knew her body would not allow.

These days, sex is not a priority for Rick and Nicole. Rick tries to hold her hand over dinner, buys flowers that are delivered to the business, but Nicole is in menopause. "I am finished with sex," she tells Rick one evening, as he is hanging Christmas lights on the back deck. That very evening, Rick tries to suggest a dip in the backyard hot tub, just as snow is beginning to fall. Nicole slams the bedroom door.

Rick gets into the warm water. It is a solo attempt at sex. He begins to pleasure himself. He takes a swig of beer, turns up the volume of his stereo surround sound. The snow falls in sync with the music. Rick tries to remember the naked women in magazines he keeps in the bottom drawer at the office. But absolutely nothing happens.

After a sleepless night next to his wife, who is also sleepless and will not speak, Rick calls a psychologist the next morning. A sex therapist. He refuses to live like this. He may not be perfect, but he has done right by his family and he works hard for everything he has. Rick will make it right by his wife Nicole, too. He has to.

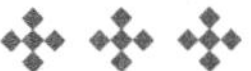

# Sheila

Sheila Ashtiju was born in Iran and then moved to America at age three. Her father Farrokh wanted the best for his family. He got his cousin to sponsor him and moved his wife and children to the United States. While Farrokh had gained a high political position in their region of Iran, he knew the toll it would take on his children to remain living there. So, he moved to Houston, Texas, and took a job running a nightclub for his cousin.

Sheila quickly learned English, as she was young and had a quick mind that could absorb just about anything that was put in front of her. She grew up speaking with a Texan twang and graduated as first in her class at Katy High School. Sheila knew many things. She knew to call herself Persian instead of Iranian. And there was a large group of Persians with whom her family was affiliated in the U.S. Sheila knew to wear the slender Prada high heels of the women in her culture. She dressed in expensive clothing; she went to the night clubs that her father now owned. There were four of them in Houston alone. And a few more in Dallas. But she only seldom drank anything with alcohol, in keeping with her Muslim religion.

Sheila applied to several medical schools. She was accepted at all of them and got almost a full ride to the University of Ohio. Her father Farrokh was not a man of many words, but when she graduated in her cap and gown, a smile grew on the right side of his mouth. Sheila then got her residency in urology back in Houston. She worked in a prominent hospital and found great monetary reward in treating patients with prostate and bladder cancer. Sheila also found enormous satisfaction in helping her patients beat the worst of odds. "I like to throw cancer on the floor and stomp on it," she said to herself in the cold Operating Room.

Sheila's life was going according to plan. Where else but in the United States could a woman have risen to such status? Her father was now immensely proud, and no longer hid his wide grin when he attended the ceremonies to award his daughter for eradicating cancer of the urinary system. After she gave a speech to the Urology Board of Texas which brought forth a standing ovation, Farrokh approached his daughter. "I have found an excellent man for you," he began. "He is in town and can meet us for dinner tomorrow night."

An arranged marriage was not uncommon in Sheila's world. Her parents had had one, and nowadays, parents of Persians still 'loosely arranged' their children for matrimony. Many of Sheila's female classmates from Katy High School in Texas were married, had children, and often had solid careers to boot. Was this a bad thing? In Sheila's logical mind, this traditional life path still made sense. She had dated a few men in college, American guys, and it had been fun.

But now, Sheila had begun a lesbian affair with a colleague. It had begun as nothing more than a make-out session on her couch after a trip to a wine bar and was now an intense and quasi-committed relationship with an oncology nurse. Her name was Stacy. Stacy was blonde, she had been a cheerleader in college for the Texas Longhorns (which made Sheila a little wary), but Stacy stood side by side with Sheila as they treated people with the kind of cancer that had once been untreatable. It was this particular work-bond that drew these women together.

Sheila nodded to her father as he offered up a potential husband for her. She knew that this was the expectation of a woman from Iran. She was supposed to have been married by age 36, not pursuing a prominent career and lusting after a blonde ex-cheerleading American. Could she ever tell her father that she was in love with a woman? No. Not without family shame. Could she throw herself into her career and abandon the possibility of a future with Stacy? Yes, but that would destroy the human she had become. Sheila knew this. She could not be the premier physician who gave radiation to bladders and prostates who *also* denied her sexuality. That would be too big a sacrifice.

There was only one choice to be made, after that evening of accolades from her fellow physicians and friends in Texas. Sheila would leave the state. She would ask Stacy to join her. She would then embark on an unusual journey into pelvic health, one that had nothing to do with surgery anymore. She would become a hormone specialist. A doctor who used science, instinct and experimentation to restore the health of sexuality.

Sheila's Persian culture valued sex for procreation; to preserve lineage and wealth, bloodlines and to keep families together. Sheila wanted no part of that. She believed in sex for the sake of sex. Because she had the requisite medical training to understand the urinary system, Sheila knew that she could expand her knowledge to the surrounding organs of the pelvis. Sheila had treated so many men with prostate problems. They came to her with concerns of cancer, but more often than not, these men had no cancer whatsoever. What these men *did* have unsatisfactory sex and urinary problems galore. These men had pain that nobody could diagnose. They described burning pain through the perineum and there were no bacteria or cancer cells to back it up.

Sheila loved sex with women. But there was a reason she had never become a gynecologist. The organs and anatomy with women were so...messy. But with men, it was cut and dry. Sheila found it easy to understand the male sex organs. God had made it straightforward for them. Until a problem occurred, and it wasn't anymore.

Sometimes people are faced with a decision that seems impossible. There are people who wallow within that impossibility for a lifetime. Sheila had vowed to herself to never become a *wallower*. She and Stacy packed their bags and moved to Pittsburgh, Pennsylvania. They got an apartment and Sheila rented an open-aired office space and painted the walls dove gray. She became a doctor who specialized in male hormones and sexual health. Dr. Ashtiju opened her own practice in the Steel City, where nobody knew her and her family was far, far away. This was her brand-new beginning.

# Oliver

Oliver was born in Alabama. His parents worked hard, his father was a white cop and his mother a Jamaican housekeeper and nanny. Oliver was biracial. And for whatever reason, this never really entered his mind. Maybe it was because he lived in a town where seeing couples of different skin color was the norm. Oliver's classmates in high school were every shade, and race was not a thing in his town.

Oliver's skin color became a thing when he decided to enlist in the United States Army just as he turned 18. His father was proud and approved of his son serving his country. But his mother, whose skin was dark and whose ancestry went back several generations on the island of Jamaica, was horrified. "I know why you are enlisting," she shouted, while vigorously scrubbing the kitchen backsplash after supper. "Because you are a black man who does not think he can do any better! What about college? You have good marks. Maybe you are not Auburn material, but you could get into State with no problem! Why in the hell are you settling for a military position? Everybody knows that minorities are the only people who go to the Middle East and die for this country nowadays!"

Oliver was confused. *Am I black?* He pondered. *And what does that have to do with wanting to get away from this old town and see the world?* Many of Oliver's friends were not going to college anyway. Instead, they signed up for jobs in manual labor and were likely going to stay in their same zip code forever. *What kind of a life is that?* The few others that were going to try college were only going to County anyway, to become paralegals or get associates degrees in business. *Where does that get anybody?*

It was an easy decision for Oliver. Despite his mother's tears and pleading, Oliver signed up for the Army and went to boot camp. He actually enjoyed awakening early, pushing his body to his physical limits. Oliver found comrades in boot camp and they also never saw him as the black man his mother insisted he was.

When he got his first M16 rifle, Oliver discovered that his abilities with a gun were second to none. He became a sharp-shooter and trained under many other snipers. It was in these moments when Oliver felt most himself, most skilled and adept as the man he was supposed to become. It felt so natural, that before Oliver boarded a flight to go to Iraq in 2004, he called his father and tried to keep the excitement out of his voice. Not that he needed to hide this from his father; but his Mom, she was a different story.

Oliver began wielding a Barrett M82 in the Middle East. He could hit a target over one mile away. While crouching in the sand in high temperatures and sleeping in a tent as the colder, desert winds swept over the dark evenings were not a walk in the park, this Alabaman man felt alive. Oliver had a gift. Often, the lieutenants and sergeants watched him while he was practice shooting. One of his higher ups even approached him one day. Oliver would never forget that moment. The sun was rising in the sky, it was likely around 11:37 am, and the scorch of high noon was on its way. The sergeant knelt next to an officer. This rarely happened in the Army. "Who taught you how to shoot like that?" The sergeant asked Oliver.

Oliver smiled, as sweat dripped down his brow. He was lucky to be able to sweat at all, given how dehydrated the soldiers had become. Oliver had heard that the soldiers from the Southern States had been sent first in Desert Storm back in 1998. This was because their bodies were acclimated to the heat they would have to endure in the desert of the Middle East. Oliver had known heat and humidity in Alabama. Maybe this was why he could sit under the blazing sun and hit any target asked of him.

Oliver returned his mind to a memory with his Dad. They had been in a field together when Oliver was only 10 years old. His father had brought him out to hunt for wild turkey. It was winter in Alabama and the men wore long sleeves. Oliver had never held a shotgun before. He had been told by his father that he could only shoot a turkey in the head. On that first day with a firearm, Oliver held up that shotgun and aimed perfectly. The turkey fell to the ground. As he and his Dad approached the dead bird, its head had been fired clean off its body.

"My Dad taught me how to shoot," Oliver replied to the sergeant, as he closed one eye, exhaled, and fired at a target so miniscule that the sergeant himself could not see it.

# Kirk

ife was good in New York City for a millennial. That is what they called Kirk and his friends. They had a title. Like Hippies, Baby Boomers or Yuppies. Kirk really did not care about the title, because he did not have many cares at all. He had moved from the suburbs of New Jersey to The Village in Manhattan. That was Greenwich Village, and anyone who knew anything called New York City "The City". Was there any other city in the world? Kirk shared a tiny apartment with three other guys. The women who slept over (and most of them didn't, it was that dirty), called it "appalling".

Kirk was a musician. He had practiced playing the drums throughout his entire adolescence. These days, he was part of a band that he believed was going someplace. While they did not have a huge following and his band did not yet have a world-wide tour, Kirk knew that it was coming. He practiced with his band in Alphabet City and felt the bass guitar notes from his band mate Pete match his snare drum with authentic synchrony.

Between some gigs with the band, Kirk tended bar to make ends meet. He didn't mind, and it was a great way to meet women. Kirk had been born tall. Height had its advantages in society. Kirk was also attractive. He knew this from the time he was in Middle School, when he was a terrible student and teachers went out of their way to help him catch up. He knew how to shrug and smirk at the world to get what he wanted.

All of this added up to a pretty sweet gig in his life. Kirk bagged tons of chicks, he had threesomes, he had women begging for repeat performances from what he perceived as mediocre one-night stands. "Sex in this city is like shooting fish in a barrel," he often scoffed to his roommates, in their "appalling" and tiny apartment.

It was all going so very well. Until Kirk began having trouble peeing. There was a fiery sensation along his urethra. He often had to sit down in order to piss, and he felt like a pussy when he was playing drums and had to use the only closed stall in the Men's bathroom. It was humiliating. The other guys in the venue had just seen him play like Taylor Hawkins for the Foo Fighters, and here Kirk was hiding in a fucking stall! To piss, not even to shit!

The pain with peeing was bad enough, but there was also a feeling of tension in his balls when he was fucking. And it only got worse when he was finished. Kirk never wanted women to stick around after a good screw, which was a good thing, because the urge to grab his balls and scream like a child was insane. He trembled and writhed alone in his twin bed after sex. He lit up his bong and smoked weed, along with shots of Maker's Mark to take the edge off the pain.

Kirk was only 24. He didn't have health insurance, nor any spare cash to go and get checked out. Kirk called his mother and made up a bullshit excuse to see a doctor. "I have a sore throat," he told her. "Maybe it is strep. I need to see a doctor in the city. Can you wire me $100 so I can get some medicine?" And his mother did just that.

Kirk could have made an appointment with an internist for his "strep throat". Instead, he went to a clinic to get tested for HIV and sexually transmitted infections. Kirk walked into a room and told the practitioner about his problems. He explained his pain with urination and sex. The doctor asked for a urine sample. Kirk explained that he would not be able to urinate for many hours, due to his excruciating pain. The doctor sent him home with a small cup, which he was instructed to fill and return as soon as possible.

He had a gig scheduled that night. But Kirk would never make it. Instead, he sat on the toilet in his apartment alone. The roommates were all out drinking, getting high, fucking women. He strained for hours to get urine in that container. Kirk hoped against all hope that he had some diagnosis for what was wrong with him. Something easily cured, like chlamydia. He finally filled the plastic cup with urine as the sun rose the next morning.

# Tom

Tom was supposed to be on an airplane to Chile. His boss had asked him to fly down and talk with a local farmer about a new red wine blend which used Merlot and Syrah grapes. This was the part of his job that Tom loved: getting to know the alchemists behind the vineyard. Especially a vineyard this small, yet up-and-coming, as this one seemed to be. A translator accompanied Tom on all his wine tastings. Nothing was more interesting than hearing about the process of how a lowly grape could become a masterpiece.

But due to Tom's new pain level (it was a pain that roiled and screeched, it never left him alone), Tom was forced to call out sick from work and take the only appointment he could get with a local urologist. As he sat in the waiting room, Tom looked around him. There were middle-aged men, a lot of them overweight. There were older men with their wives, bickering behind magazines about the long wait in the office and the rising cost of healthcare services. Tom wondered if his problem was unique. He was now unable to sit for longer than three minutes and declined his wife's advances after date night. His crotch was killing him.

Tom was ushered into a private treatment room and instructed by a young and peppy nurse to take off his clothes and put on a hospital gown. He had endured the requisite finger in the ass for annual exams by his Primary Care Physician and knew that this would likely be part of today's spectacle. Tom stood in the cold and sterile room as his brow twitched in pain.

The urologist entered and shook Tom's hand. He was a young guy, maybe in his late twenties. What would compel a person to want to spend thousands of dollars on medical school to treat dicks, Tom wondered? The guy seemed nice enough, though, and began with a lengthy interview about Tom's symptoms.

As Tom described how his problem had begun, starting with a small gnawing ache in his penis over two years ago, leading up to the escalation of his rectal spasms and avoidance of sex because of the intense pain it elicited, the urologist merely nodded. Tom continued, he began a full-throttle rant, one he had not known was within him, and told the doctor how his groin was ruining his career, his marriage, and the very life that he had once enjoyed.

After Tom was finished with his full-throttle rant, the urologist asked him to bend over and performed a routine prostate check. "Your prostate is somewhat enlarged," the young kid with the medical degree declared. *How could you possibly know this? Didn't you just finish your residency ten months ago? How many prostates have you touched in that span of time?* But Tom said none of this out loud. He was instructed to get back into his clothing and wait for the boy doctor to return to the room.

The young doctor came back into the treatment room, his attitude confident and bordering on cocky. "You have prostatitis," the urologist stated with authority. That was the diagnosis.

"What does that mean?" Tom asked the doctor.

"It means that there is an inflammatory response in your prostate gland," he replied. "It could be due to an infection within that organ. And your prostate in right next to your rectum, so this could account for the rectal spasms you've been having."

Tom was dumbfounded. An infection in his prostate? From what? From where? Tom had only had a few girlfriends before his wife, and he was a stickler for condom use back then.

"How do you know there is an infection in my prostate?" Tom countered. "Is there a test you can do to determine that?"

"I will need a semen sample to confirm the bacteria. You need to rely on my experience here," the doctor answered. "I see this problem every day. Most guys don't want to talk about it, but they come here with exactly the same symptoms that you are describing."

The doctor was finishing up. He pulled out a prescription pad. "I am going to give you an antibiotic. I want you to take it for one month. I am also prescribing you some oral steroids for the pain. Take these in a five-day course before a long trip overseas. But you cannot rely on these to control your pain. The side-effects for steroids are bad and I have faith that the antibiotics will help you. Come back to me in one month."

Tom got into his BMW and wanted to punch the steering wheel. He had cancelled a trip to Chile for this? *To be told that he had a nebulous infection in his prostate and to be given antibiotics?* Tom drove home to his wife and daughters. They sat at dinner, eating duck confit, and chatted about school plays and soccer and the perils of Algebra II. Tom looked up at his wife. Her face fell with what looked like pity. She knew that Tom was far away, in a place he never spoke of. The truth of the matter was that Tom was planning on staying away. Because there was no reason to drag his wife and best friend down with him. Silence was the only way.

# Rick

It is now springtime in Pittsburgh. Which means that the snow has melted, the skies are still overcast, and the temperature sometimes gets above 50 degrees. Rick's business is booming, and he realizes he needs to hire new plumbers. He does not mind this, as his son Francis will be going to college in the fall. Yes, Francis will be the first man in the family to get a university degree. Rick is immensely proud, and he helps his son choose between the multiple colleges to which Francis has shown interest.

Rick's wife Nicole can barely get out of bed. Even since she put a moratorium on sex last December, she has been slowly sinking into a major depressive episode. Nicole suffers from intense migraines, muscle and joint pain and insomnia. While Rick had thought that going to a sex therapist might spice things up between them, he attends exactly three sessions of sex therapy alone. There now seems no reason to continue without the presence of his wife.

Rick spends hours on the Internet as he tries to find a solution for his wife Nicole's new despair. She is not receptive to treatment ideas for menopause, and Rick is not going to push it. Their regular, daily fighting has now dimmed to a mere complacency; they are now roommates, though Rick performs all the household chores, grocery shopping and even does the books for his wife at the business. He has become a single parent to Francis. Nicole barely gets into the shower and sleeps in the master bedroom, while Rick takes residence in the basement.

In a fit of desperation, Rick orders testosterone supplements. If his wife cannot assist him in any type of sex, he might as well be able to get a hard-on and watch some porn. What harm could it do? A life without sex is a life not worth living. It is bad enough that Rick must assume the role of the woman in the family. But to run a business, bring home all the money and be a good father to Francis is really wearing on Rick.

Rick gets a phone call from one of his clients. He has not been to this client's particular location and sent one of his new plumbers to do a renovation for a doctor's office out in Sewickley. The doctor has personally called him, after paying the full bill *in cash* to ask for another favor. "I need another bathroom in a remote corner of my office. Could you please come by and tell me what it would cost to add it?" Rick agrees and tells the doctor he can come by her office tomorrow morning at 10 to give her an estimate.

He arrives the next day, after driving through what seems like sleet falling from the sky in April. It is a well-appointed office, Rick thinks. A woman comes out from behind the glass enclosure of the front desk. She introduces herself as Sheila. This woman is smoking hot. She has long, dark hair and what would seem to be a fantastic body under her woolen sweater.

"We spoke on the phone last night," Sheila explains." I will show you where I want to add another bathroom. The work you and your men do is excellent, by the way. I am from Houston and getting a good contractor down there is damn near impossible." *Is Sheila the doctor?* Rick wonders. He has never seen a doctor look this good.

Rick assesses the room, takes measurements and checks out the plumbing in the rest of the office, to ensure that he can create a small bathroom where the doctor wants it. "This won't be cheap or easy, but I can do it," he tells her.

Rick and Sheila agree on a price. She crosses her arms during the negotiation. There is something tough about her, something that tells Rick that this woman is not to be crossed. Sheila reminds Rick of his wife Nicole, when she was young and negotiated buying a beautiful house for the two of them, refusing to pay a penny more than it was worth. Nicole had looked so sexy in that moment, staring down the realtor with a ferocity and intention that struck fear in most men. Instead, Rick had found it the sexiest thing he had ever seen. Where had that woman gone? Into a bed, with knotted hair, black circled-eyes and barely the will to breathe.

As Rick leaves the office, feeling something akin to arousal (even though he has not had a full-on erection in months), he turns back. There is a row of brochures. One advertises help for enlarged prostates. The next is for something called "platelet rich plasma", for hair loss. Whoever heard of such a thing? It is that last brochure that catches Rick's eye. *Erectile Dysfunction: A Holistic Guide for Every Man.*

Rick snatches up the brochure and shoves it into his breast pocket. After getting through a thirteen-hour workday, Rick descends into the basement with a can of Pabst Blue Ribbon. He reads the brochure from cover to cover. *I am not the only guy in the world who has this,* he thinks. *There are people who can help me. There is someone very specific who can help me. Her name is Sheila.*

But how was Rick going to talk to such a gorgeous female creature about his limp dick?

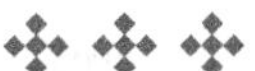

# Sheila

Dr. Sheila Ashtiju had begun her practice in Pittsburgh. While it was a cash-based business (Dr. Ashtiju did not take insurance plans, her services were "out of network"), she had no shortage of patients coming to her for pelvic problems. Maybe this was because she opened her practice in Sewickley, one of the ritziest suburbs in the Steel City. The people in this area had lots of disposable income. But a more likely reason why Sheila was so sought after was because men whose sex lives were deemed inadequate by themselves were quite likely to do something about it, even if that meant spending hundreds of dollars on injections, hormone creams and vitamin supplements.

What Dr. Ashtiju did not realize was that she was an excellent physician for this patient population. Her expertise in dealing with prostate cancer had given her a very unique skill set to figure out the driving cause behind most sexual, urinary and bowel dysfunctions. All these things needed to happen in this small area of the pelvis. While Dr. Ashtiju missed getting in there with a scalpel, she found herself amazed by the way the testicles hung neatly encased in the scrotal sack. When she first examined each man she treated, she had him stand while she sat on a stool. With gloved fingers, she palpated the testes. Were they symmetrical? Was one testis significantly larger than the other? She then moved her fingers up to the epididymis, the tiny coil located above each testis. The epidid-ymis housed the sperm and felt like a miniscule ball of steel wool covered in flannel. Dr. Ashtiju followed the swooping de-scent of the spermatic cord on each side of the scrotum. Was there scar tissue? Was one of the cords bound down to the tissues beneath it? Finally, she assessed the scrotal skin for turgidity. Was it elastic and rubbery, or was it thin and fragile?

It was a fantastic way to make a living. Sheila was able to take her time with each of her patients because she knew she would be adequately compensated. By not having to deal with insurance companies, she saved herself hours of paperwork and a mountain of headaches. There were the occasional weir-dos who were attracted to her and believed she was touching their balls for fun; but those guys were few and far between, and Sheila was able to stop them cold with just a level-headed gaze. They either never came back to her office or ceased with the "hot for my dick doctor" bullshit.

Things were going so well. Except that Sheila had no sex drive whatsoever. Her girlfriend Stacy was working at the University of Pittsburgh and had scads of new friends. Stacy often begged Sheila to go out with them to the North Side, but Sheila preferred to stay at home on the couch. When Stacy did return home in an Uber and after three dirty martinis, she was starving for sex. Sheila went through the motions but could not orgasm.

Was it because she was gazing at scrotal sacks all day? She did not think so. The male anatomy had never turned her on. Dr. Sheila had a few theories on why her sexual drive had recently tanked. Firstly, she had moved from sunny Houston all the way to Western Pennsylvania. The weather in Pittsburgh rivaled that of Seattle, Washington, in terms of cloudy days.

Only Pittsburgh was frigidly cold in the winter, with inches of ice lining the sidewalks for months. Surely, she was suffering from Seasonal Affective Disorder due to lack of sunlight.

Secondly, Sheila had left her entire family behind. She called her parents every day en route to work, after scraping off the ice from the windshield of her Mercedes. Her father Farrokh had not understood her reason for moving. "You were doing so well down here," he told his daughter in Farsi. Sheila had been doing well in the work and status department, that much was true. Yet she consistently felt that she was living a lie, in not being able to come out as a lesbian and bring Stacy to family dinners.

The move had been much harder than Sheila could ever had imagined. Pittsburgh was a cool city, but that did not change the fact that it always takes work to start over. Moving and changing jobs were two of the biggest stressors in life, everyone knew that. But Sheila understood hormones better than most endocrinologists. She understood the delicate interplay of the thyroid with the menstrual cycle.

After performing a series of blood work and a testing her saliva on the nineteenth day of her cycle, Sheila discovered that her adrenal glands were barely working. There was simply no cortisol in her bloodstream. And it was cortisol and the adrenal glands that synthesized the sex hormones, progesterone and testosterone. With burnt-out adrenals, it came as no surprise that Sheila could not climax and had no interest in sex. This was the body's evolutionary way of protecting women from pregnancy during times of famine and moving across the prairie. When the body had spent up its stores for Fight or Flight after prolonged and protracted stress, there was no cortisol in the bloodstream anymore. Without cortisol, there was no progesterone secreted around the time of ovulation. Without progesterone, there was zero desire for sex. The body had bigger fish to fry.

There was nothing that could be done about this, back on the prairie. But now was a different story! Sheila prescribed herself progesterone cream. She rubbed it into her forearms and the backs of her knees from day 14 to day 26 of her menstrual cycle. She applied compounded testosterone cream to her vulva three nights a week. She also took a supplement: it was the adrenal gland of a grass-fed bison, ground up and placed into a little capsule.

Why was she doing this? Sheila was building her body back up, after the biggest loss she had ever sustained. She was only 36 years old. She refused to spend the rest of her years as a woman who did not enjoy sex. Because that is precisely why she had opened her clinic in the first place, so that people could find their fullest sexual potential! Dr. Sheila Ashtiju would show the city of Pittsburgh exactly what she was made of. And she would do this with the former cheerleader of the Texas Longhorns at her side.

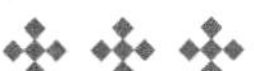

# Oliver

Oliver's Dad had been diagnosed with prostate cancer while his son was overseas in the Army. Oliver had been worried, but his father assured him that everything would be fine. "They have this new treatment available," his father said. "They can put these radioactive seeds in the groin, and they get rid of the cancer. I won't have to get my prostate removed. Don't come home for this, son. Stay where you are. If you come back here for my treatment, it will only worry your mother. She will try to convince you to be an Alabama boy again. And there is nothing for you here. Your decision to leave was a good one."

Still, Oliver worried for months about his Dad. He kept his mind on his tour in Afghanistan. About ten months after this conversation with his father, Oliver received another phone call from him. "You are not going to believe this, Ollie! I am cured of prostate cancer! Everything is back to normal. It is like nothing was ever wrong!" Oliver exhaled the longest breath of his life. In shooting, inhalation happens when the target is lined up. Then, with the finger on the trigger and one eye on the scope, the shooter exhales and shifts his body forward into the line of aim. Exhalation is the moment when the target is perfectly clear. Especially for a sharpshooter. Everything was really going to be okay.

When Oliver boarded a plane that Thanksgiving to return to the States, he felt nostalgia. An aching, longing feeling of home washed over him. As he strode through the Montgomery Airport in his Army fatigues, he became aware of the looks of respect from civilians. Gone were the days of disdain for the military. Oliver had done something with his life. He had done something significant.

The turkey dinner that year was fantastic. Oliver missed his mother's cooking, of okra, baked pumpkin from the garden, and warm pone (a dessert native to the islands of the Caribbean). His father was beaming over the table. Afterwards, the men watched football together on the couch. They drank beer and said nothing; there was nothing to be said. It was just one of those idyllic moments, just as the turkey hunting had been when Oliver had discovered his most sought-after ability to shoot a gun when he was merely a ten-year-old boy.

Later that night, Oliver went to a local tavern. He did not wear his fatigues, as he believed that to be begging for compliments. Oliver didn't need any compliments tonight. He needed his old buddies. There they sat, lined up at the bar. They pounded his back as they hugged him. They bought him shots of Crown Royal. That evening had the warmth of a home-coming bonfire.

What made it even more sweet a welcoming was a hot chick named Talulah. She raised one eyebrow from across the bar and Oliver introduced himself. They had sex in the front cab of his pickup truck later that night. It was this sequence of unraveling events which were hurtling Oliver irrevocably towards his destiny.

Less than one year after that Thanksgiving homecoming, Oliver had moved back to Alabama. He secured a job as a State Trooper. He married Talulah and they bought a house in a very nice section of town. Oliver went to that same tavern where he had met her, but only once a month now. He realized that his high school comrades were all sloppy drunks. They were hell-bent on getting a break from their wives and kids. After only two beers at the tavern, Oliver drove home to his wife. They laughed as they showered together. Then they had phenomenal sex.

Oliver slept beautifully every night. In his dreams, he held his sniper's rifle and fired his gun as an expert would. It had all been worth it. The trip to Iraq, then Afghanistan, the desert heat, the shitty food, the poor living conditions of being in the Middle East had all been worth it. Because all of that had brought him to this moment right now.

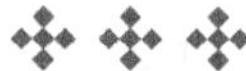

# Kirk

I n the thick of his most agonizing discomfort, Kirk had returned to the clinic which tested him for Sexually Transmitted Infections. The doctor had run every single test in the book, including an HIV test. Kirk was negative for everything. He did not have a urinary tract infection (they are unusual in men, the doctor explained, due to the length of the male urethra). This pain was awful, peeing felt like acid creeping out through the tip of his penis, but Kirk just kept going. There were nights that he played in the band and simply got rip-roaring drunk to shut out the noise in his crotch. That merely led to a wicked hangover and worsening of his piss problem the next day.

But then something strange happened. As quickly as the pain had begun, it mysteriously stopped. Kirk had done nothing different, except that he had avoided sex because it was not worth the horror of the climax. He had even stopped masturbating, and his sex drive dwindled down to nothing. When he awoke in the morning, he didn't have a hard-on. Instead, he felt nothing in his pelvis. It was an empty and silent thing, this absence of pain. Kirk did not trust it at first. He continued to pee sitting down, which had been one thing that helped him when his symptoms were most severe.

Days wore on, and the pain receded into the distance like a bad dream. This shocked Kirk. He kept waiting for that knock on the door, that reminder of how bad things were going to get.

Instead, there was another knock. It was a phone call from a music producer who wanted to sponsor Kirk and his band to do a nationwide tour.

Kirk bought a new drum set. The band practiced every night in the studio. Nobody drank any booze, and Kirk curtailed his pot smoking to only a few times weekly. There was something about marijuana which helped him with whole-body relaxation. He took a few hits from his joint and felt his mind declutter. This, in turn, also helped Kirk to connect more to his music. There was a new focus to the band, a new purity to their sound. They seemed to be playing with one soul.

Kirk and his roommates cleaned out their disgusting apartment. Kirk had a few one-night stands before he left Manhattan. Nothing off-the-chain awesome, but it was sex without pain, and Kirk would take that. He felt himself getting hard in the mornings again. He peed standing up. Kirk went for daily runs to clear his head before the tour. Up and down the East Side, just the pounding of his Saucony's on the pavement and the hum of the city all around him.

By the time that the tour began, and the guys played cards on a bus which rolled through the Midwest, things were looking up. The band was gathering a following. The music was building momentum. Kirk forgot that he had ever had that pain. It was like a nightmare of childhood; the kind of haunting dream that only visits the young mind of a boy. And Kirk had grown up. There was nothing that could slow him down now.

# Tom

Tom had taken the dubious advice of his urologist. The medical treatment for prostatitis was to take many types of antibiotics in separate courses to determine which strain of bacteria was infesting his prostate. Tom faithfully swallowed these pills and waited for a change in his symptoms. But a change never came. Tom was forced to go on international flights while he cried in the bathroom. It was humiliating how this pain had taken over his life.

Tom had nowhere to turn. Until one day, after scouring the Internet for solutions, he happened upon the name of a physician who specialized in pelvic pain. There were symptoms described in bullet points (pain with urination, rectal spasms, constipation, pain on arousal and ejaculation), and Tom had every single one of them. This doctor worked out of Hoboken, a happening New Jersey city outside of Manhattan. Because Tom was forever in airports for plane layovers in New York City, he called the doctor and made an appointment. There was a six-month waiting list, but this was worth waiting for.

Tom finally arrived in the office of Dr. Nathan Shah. The doctor's presence was calm and unflustered. He asked Tom numerous questions about the type of pain he was experiencing and the activities which triggered them. "It is so difficult to know what triggers my symptoms these days," Tom replied. "The pain used to wax and wane, but it is now constant.

I cannot do anything to make it go away." The doctor nodded solemnly.

"You have what we call 'Chronic Pelvic Pain Syndrome'", Dr Shah explained. "Many men have it, they just don't want to tell anyone. And there are very few practitioners who can get to the source of it. Most urologists diagnose it as 'prostatitis', and they administer antibiotics to patients like you. But there is not enough evidence in the medical literature to suggest that this pain is caused by an active infection. Which is why the antibiotics rarely work on patients like you."

Tom felt like he had just hit a grand slam in Fenway Park when the Red Sox were down at the end of the World Series. Finally! There was someone who understood what he was talking about! There was a reason for this suffering. It had a name. And, as Tom would soon find out, there was a way to treat it.

The treatment for this condition would require a series of injections in Tom's groin. It would span over six weeks, one injection per week. Tom would have to go to Hoboken to get these injections, which was far from Rhode Island. And medical insurance did not cover this treatment. It was expensive. "This is a huge undertaking," Dr. Shah counseled. "But for those with symptoms as severe as the ones you are describing, it offers tremendous relief."

Tom nodded and smiled, for the first time in months. He agreed to have his bloodwork taken and set up an appointment for his first injection in two weeks. "In addition to the treatment I can offer you, there are some lifestyle adjustments I want to suggest," Dr. Shah advised. "If you do not change the way you are living your life, these injections may not help. I want to suggest meditation. Before you laugh, there are some great apps on your phone that you can try. Secondly, I want you to engage in some type of exercise daily. Try to avoid running or bike riding. They can irritate your symptoms. But activities like walking or yoga will calm you down and allow you to get some more sleep at night."

These things were all very doable for Tom. He felt a tight coil in his chest unravel as he listened to Dr. Nathan Shah. "Do you smoke?" The doctor asked. Tom shook his head no. "Do you drink alcohol?" Tom explained his job title as a sommelier. "Abstaining from alcohol for the time being would be suggested. However, given your line of work, that may not be possible. Please limit your wine drinking to work purposes, only," the doctor replied. Tom laughed, which elicited a grin from the doctor. "Never before have I given the instruction to drink solely on the job," Dr. Shah remarked wryly.

"There is one final thing I need you to look into," Dr. Shah concluded. "I want you to get some physical therapy for this condition."

"Excuse me if I sound obtuse, but how could a physical therapist help with my problem?" Tom asked, confounded.

Dr Nathan Shah nodded and replied. "Every patient tells me this. Until they go to a physical therapist who specializes in the pelvic floor. These PT's believe that the muscles of your perineum are causing some of the pain you have been experiencing. Trust me, I was as doubtful about this as you look right now. But I have sent quite a few patients to pelvic floor physical therapy, and I am seeing some great and powerful results. You should be able to find one of these practitioners up in Rhode Island. Coupled with the injections, you stand an even greater chance of full recovery if you do this type of physical therapy as well."

Tom felt renewed. There was something jaunty in his step as he walked through the streets of Hoboken. He had been toying with going to a local wine bar before heading back to the airport. Instead, he rented a car and drove directly home to his family. It took over 5 hours with traffic. But that beat sitting on another airplane. Besides, there was something very important that he had to tell his wife Casey.

Tom entered his home and the lights were out. His daughters were asleep in their rooms with the doors closed. Tom entered the room of his wife and leaned over to kiss her mouth. As she stirred to awaken, Tom removed his tie. He began to speak. There were so many words. There was so much to tell this woman, a woman who had become certain that her husband was an alcoholic or a cheater or both. Casey's eyes widened. Tom knew exactly what she now realized. *This is why he will not have sex with me. This is why he stays up all night drinking wine. This is why I thought he would leave me and the girls forever.*

While that evening did not end in penetrative sex, Casey moaned in ecstasy and Tom knew that he might be able to return to the life that he once knew.

# Rick

Rick didn't know what to expect from his first visit with Dr. Sheila Ashtiju. He sat in her waiting room and filled out a lengthy questionnaire. The section about Rick's health habits was a no-brainer: he knew that he was overweight, that his diet was garbage and that he had not exercised in years. After writing all of this down, he moved on to the next section of the form.

1. How many times per week do you climax?
2. What kinds of sex do you engage in: manual, oral, vaginal, anal?
3. Do you have a sexual partner(s)? If so, how many?
4. How often do you masturbate?
5. Do you require pornography to ejaculate?
6. How long does it typically take you to reach a climax?
7. Are you able to get an erection sufficient enough for penetrative sex? If so, are you able to continue with sex until climax?

This was downright humiliating! Rick felt sweat bead along his forehead. He glanced around the waiting room to see if anyone else seemed as anxious as he felt. There were only two other people in the room; one was an older man in his seventies, who had clearly just come from the gym. He was a lean silver fox. It made sense that an old man would need to come to this office. The other person in the waiting room was a woman in her late thirties. What was she doing here? Rick was under the impression that this office treated only men. Perhaps she was the girlfriend of a guy who couldn't get it up either. (Rick clung to this hope. Yes, maybe guys in their thirties had the same problem that he did. Maybe he wasn't alone. After all, Dr. Ashtiju had a waiting list of several months to see her. Rick had waited quite some time to get his appointment. Maybe erectile dysfunction was like the common cold).

Before the privacy consent form at the end of the paperwork, there was another round of questioning that Rick found odd. Rick felt some embarrassment in writing down that he was only masturbating to porn, that there was no sex with his wife and there hadn't been for years; but that seemed like important information for a sex doctor. Yeah, that all made sense. But now there were questions about other "life stressors": Was Rick going through financial troubles? Bankruptcy? Was he taking care of elderly parents? Was he in a satisfying relationship? Had he moved in the last year? Was he going through a divorce? Were his children healthy and well-adjusted?

Rick wrote nothing down in this section. His business was expanding, and he often had to turn away work. His parents were both deceased, so he was not caring for them. Francis was going to college next year, and Rick was extremely proud of his son. Rick had lived in the same house for over twenty years. And his marriage to Nicole had been stable throughout that time.

Rick was ushered into a treatment room by one of the front desk girls. He was instructed to undress and put on a gown, with the opening in the back. He tried on the gown and it was far too small for him. Rick leaned against the treatment table, his socked feet crossed, trying with all his might to seem nonchalant; like a guy playing pool, resting one hip against the pool table, until it was his turn to shoot next.

Dr. Ashtiju entered the treatment room. She was far more beautiful than Rick had remembered. She wore a white lab coat that was cinched at the waist. The doctor shook his hand and remained standing during the beginning of the treatment session. She had a way of making Rick feel at ease. After a few minutes, he was standing with his feet apart, his hands clasped in front of him, and he no longer felt like a poser in a pool hall.

Dr. Ashtiju perched herself on a high stool and typed into a computer, while she made sure to look at him while she questioned him. "When would you say that you first noticed that your erections were inadequate to your liking?"

Rick had to ponder this. "I never really thought about it, I guess," he replied. "Maybe about four to five years ago."

Dr. Ashtiju typed that into her computer. "And what happened four to five years ago in your life? Was there a trauma of some sort? A change in your job? The death of a loved one?"

Now Rick was completely perplexed. *What was this woman getting at? That his erectile dysfunction was somehow HIS OWN FAULT? That his dick was at the whim of anything that could possibly go wrong in his life? Shit happens to everyone! That is just fucking reality...*And then it hit him. It was exactly five years ago when his wife Nicole began to stay in bed all day. She no longer did the bookkeeping for his business. She stopped cleaning the house and showered only twice a week. Over the span of the last half of a decade, Nicole's life had become smaller and smaller. She did not take care of her own son. Granted, Francis was only 12 years old back then, and 12-year-old boys are pretty self-sufficient. But still…she had stopped packing his lunches, helping him with homework and going to his soccer games. Rick had taken up the slack for all of that.

When the words finally came out, Rick could not stop talking for several minutes. The doctor merely sat and listened. She was not typing in her computer anymore. Rick felt something uncoil in his stomach. This quiet disappointment that he had held so close was now leaving his body. Never had he told anyone the things that he told Dr. Sheila Ashtiju that day.

When all the words had been said, from the man that had held up his family for so long, Dr. Ashtiju did an examination of Rick's penis and testicles. It did not feel weird, her poking around while sitting on a stool in front of him as he stood in his undersized treatment gown. She then arose, removed her gloves and brought out a clipboard. She wrote things down and handed Rick a piece of paper. Her handwriting was rather legible, for a doctor's.

"Here is where I want to begin with you," Dr. Ashtuji said. "I am going to do some bloodwork. I suspect that your cortisol is low. This is because the kind of stress you have been under for the past few years would likely tap out your adrenal glands." She showed Rick a picture of a man's abdomen and pelvis. "The adrenal glands sit on top of your kidneys. They produce cortisol, which is the 'fight or flight' chemical. Because you have been in the 'fight or flight' mode by taking care of everyone around you, your adrenals are tired and cannot produce the cortisol you need to get aroused. I want you to take a few vitamin supplements to build up your adrenals again."

Rick was confused. Before he could ask, *what about some Viagra,* the doctor continued talking. "Hear me out next. It is cortisol that is required to make testosterone. Once we improve your cortisol production, your body can synthesize more testosterone to improve arousal on its own. In the meantime, I am going to prescribe testosterone cream. It should be applied to your scrotum every night before bed. In time, you will notice more rigid erections with this treatment plan." *More rigid erections,* Rick thought. *Now we are talking!*

"Finally, I am going to ask you to try and lose some weight," Dr. Ashtiju suggested. "This is not a judgment about you or your lifestyle choices. I am merely pointing out what science has shown: the more belly weight that pushes down through the pelvis, the more challenging it is for the penis to achieve the fully erect, or stiff position that is required for more pleasurable sex."

Rick nodded in assent. His primary doctor had suggested weight loss programs and diets for the last several years. Rick was told that his A1C levels were high and that he was at risk for diabetes because he was overweight. But with everything else pressing on his mind, Rick did not care about the future possibility of diabetes. However, if weight loss could help Rick to be able to have sex again, then he would certainly try a diet.

A few weeks later, Rick noticed that he had more energy throughout the day. He could sleep through the night. He walked three miles a day, rain or shine (although it was usually rain or snow in Pittsburgh). Rick took a supplement made from a cow's adrenal gland, which had been dehydrated and pulverized into a small brown capsule. Each night, he used a cotton swab to coat his balls with white testosterone cream. While he did not notice that much change in his erections, he had lost twenty pounds. More women looked his way as he stood in line at the Giant Eagle. Things were looking up.

# Sheila

Sheila never knew exactly when it was that she realized she was a lesbian. There had been a friend in high school. They were partners in chemistry lab. Her name was Emily and she had red hair and one of those Irish noses that turned up at the end. Both teenagers were obsessed with getting good grades. They both wanted to get into Med School; they had been given the gift of that early longing for their future craft, while most others in high school were floundering with what to do with themselves after age 18.

Emily and Sheila were competitive by nature, though strangely, as the top two science students at Katy High School, they did not compete against each other. Mixing liquids over Bunsen burners was their silent companionable activity. Side by side, these two girls were never far apart. Before big exams, they sat in the library until it closed. Then, the two girls would go to one another's homes to continue to study throughout the night. Usually, Emily went to Sheila's house, as Farrokh was protective and did not want his Persian daughter sleeping overnight in an American's home. However, when Sheila's grandmother died and her parents had to fly back to Iran, her father requested that Sheila stay at Emily's home for one week, so that she would not be alone and unsupervised in the house.

It was the week before Christmas and the two girls had just passed their midterms with flying colors. They sat underneath

Emily's tree and sipped eggnog (this was not the kind with alcohol, but the thick kind from the convenience store. Sheila had never tasted anything more delicious). Emily's family lived in an enormous and sprawling mansion. Emily practically had an entire wing of the house to herself. Emily's parents went to bed at 11. The girls stayed up until midnight and then went to Emily's bedroom.

They laughed as they washed their faces, applied prescription acne medication (rich girls in Houston *always* saw doctors to ensure perfect skin) and brushed their teeth. They got under the sheets in sweatpants and T shirts. Sheila never knew who started it. It felt completely mutual. Emily's mouth was on Sheila's, their tongues danced together. The two girls wrapped their arms around each other.

Sheila had French kissed boys before. But she had never felt this hot sweetness between her legs. As they kissed further and removed their shirts, Sheila was worried that she would wet the bed with her juices. Emily climbed on top of her and began to writhe her hips on top of Sheila's. The outpouring of liquid continued with this friction and Sheila wanted to scream with pleasure. But she didn't.

The next morning, Sheila awoke shirtless and alone in Emily's bed. Sheila got dressed and went down to the kitchen. Emily was smug and distant, playing up to her mother who was making banana pancakes, in a way that teenagers usually don't. Sheila knew in that second that their friendship was over. There would be no more afternoons in the chemistry lab, no more all-nighters of cramming for tests. What made things even worse was when Emily began to compete against Sheila in science contests.

One year later, when Sheila went to college, she only dated men. She enjoyed being courted by men, the silly pretenses of having a car door opened, a chair pulled out at an expensive restaurant where she would never be allowed to open her wallet or pay for dinner. This dance of chivalry in modern times reminded Sheila of her parents. Their marriage had been arranged and Farrokh and her mother still lived by these archaic, yet artfully constructed set of rules.

Sheila enjoyed this act of dating men until it came to intimacy. When men kissed her in their Acuras after a three-course dinner, their lips were coarse, their tongues messy and aggressive. When they reached under her shirt to tweak her nipples, Sheila needed to keep from audibly wincing. And the sex? It was always the same. They took her to the bedrooms of their dorms and apartments, she lay on her back and they rammed her ferociously for a few minutes until they moaned and expelled their ejaculate into a condom.

It wasn't until her urology residency that Sheila met Stacy. Stacy was bubbly, so very damned American. She had a dimpled face, blonde hair that was always styled to perfection and a heart-shaped ass, which Sheila noticed despite Stacy's uniform of hospital scrubs. After a grueling night in the Operating Room Stacy invited Sheila out for a drink. They went to a wine bar. Stacy ordered Moscato, Sheila, a glass of Cabernet. Despite her fatigue from having just removed a prostate and part of a patient's bladder, it was not lost on Sheila that this nurse was intermittently touching her. She began by just brushing Sheila's hand with her manicured fingers when she was animatedly talking. This progressed to Stacy's hand on Sheila's knee.

As they walked back to their cars, no words were spoken. Sheila got into the car of this blonde American nurse and was driven to Stacy's apartment. Stacy unlocked her front door, pulled Sheila inside and their mouths met in the darkness. A short while later, Sheila lay naked on a living room carpet. In dim candlelight, she watched as Stacy leaned over her, her nipples brushing Sheila's own. Stacy teased Sheila for over an hour, touching and licking her everywhere but the place she craved the most.

When Sheila finally came, the carpet beneath her was drenched. Stacy returned from between Sheila's legs, kissed her slowly on her mouth, and whispered, *"Wasn't that worth waiting for?"*

The next morning, they made a breakfast of spinach omelets, took a bath together and continued that which had unquestionably been worth waiting for.

# Kirk

Being part of a band had a lot of perks. Kirk was smart enough to take the multiple sex offers from young hot groupies and then be able to shut out the bullshit. There was no future with these women. There were no consequences to the playtime of being a musician. While the guys were on tour on the bus, there was heavy drinking during the day. When they arrived at certain cities, they all had access to every drug imaginable. And because they were young, these boys had boundless energy. Kirk could awaken from a night of sex and snorting coke and play at his best when they arrived at the next destination.

The band tour was hitting a few glitches, however. In Omaha, Nebraska, there had been an outbreak of young guys in the mosh pit at the venue during their final song. One of the concert goers had wielded a gun. After the cops came and an investigation was done, it was determined that the gun had no bullets in it. But that did not prevent utter tumult during the band's final number, and it was Kirk's favorite song to play on the drums.

It was that night in Omaha that changed things. And Kirk had no idea why. He got along with the other band members. Kirk was playing solidly; he had never really fucked up on stage. Not like Pete the bass guitarist had, when he stumbled off the stage and vomited during one of their gigs. Being on tour was a really good time. All Kirk had to do was to fool around with drugs and women in the off hours and play as he knew how to do when asked. Playing the drums felt like being a kid to Kirk. His mother had gotten him drum lessons when he was four years old. Kirk remembered the shouting of his father through the paper-thin walls of their house. "What made you think you could spend $30 of my hard-earned money to buy drum lessons for that nitwit? He can't even fucking read, but you think it is important that he plays a musical instrument? Are you fucking that drum teacher, is that it, Arlene? Is that why you want these lessons for Kirk?"

This was followed by his mother's pleas to keep his father calm. Which was then followed by Kirk's father storming into the kitchen and pouring four fingers of Wild Turkey into the same glass that was served to the child with orange juice every morning. Kirk's Dad smoked in the house. Kirk never found this odd and his father had Camel Cash. This meant that his father bought enough Camel cigarettes to gain points which became actual hoodies, posters and neon signs advertising the cigarettes within their home. Kirk's Dad was very proud of his Camel Cash and the objects that they earned him.

This sort of argument between his parents persisted every single night until Kirk turned 10. It was on one sunny afternoon that Kirk walked home from school when he found his mother sobbing in his father's Lazy Boy. "Your father is gone," Kirk's mother said, with mucous dripping down her nose, as she slurped from one of the Camel cigarettes from a leftover pack. That was all Kirk's Dad had left behind; a half a pack of Camels.

Kirk did not remember much of those years, from the time his father left to around the time he turned 15. During that time, Kirk's mother worked two jobs. She began her day at K Mart and then worked the evening shift as a motel receptionist. She came home after Kirk had fallen asleep. He remembered that she came into his room and kissed his forehead, while he pretended to be asleep.

It was during those years that Kirk really learned to play the drums. He had nothing left to lean on. His Dad was gone, and his mother might as well of been. Kirk went to school, got mediocre grades (he was a C-type of student), went to play drums in the school music room for as long as time permitted after school, and got a job pumping gasoline at a local station. The owner of the gas station was named Ivan. He was Russian and built like a giant bear. Ivan often brought Kirk plates of warm food that his elderly mother had prepared. "Here," the Russian said, as he thrust a plate towards Kirk. "Eat before your shift starts. It looks like nobody is feeding you at home."

After ravenously eating food which tasted like it was made for royalty, Kirk went out in the cold in Garfield, NJ, and filled the gas tanks of people who said nothing to him. This was okay with Kirk, as he was accustomed to only two kinds of noise: the shouting of his father, long gone, and the thumping of a drumbeat. The silence was welcome in his young, teenaged life. Kirk went home at night, his hands smelling of cash and gasoline. He left $50 on his mother's kitchen table each week, to help to pay his way. His mother never mentioned the money, she had never asked for it. It was just an unspoken rule that Kirk was supposed to pay for being alive. So, he did.

It was not until the tour was in full-swing and the Omaha incident occurred that Kirk's pain returned. That searing, horrible pain in his crotch. He noticed that he had premature ejaculation with the hot groupies; this had never happened before.

Peeing was an exercise in torture and sitting on the stool of the drum set was horrendous. Kirk did whatever he could to keep the pain at bay. Oxycodone helped, and these pills were offered and available at least 50% of the time on tour. Booze made the pain go away while Kirk was drinking, but the pain which coupled his hangover was unbearable.

It was not all bad, though. Through the lull of his hours on tour with the band, Kirk rediscovered a memory of his father when he had been happily drunk. There were times when his Dad came home and was in a good mood. He kissed Kirk's mother on the lips and sat with Kirk in the living room on the sectional sofa. The smell of Camel cigarettes filled the air. His Dad played a CD of the Eagles. "Listen to me, son. Some people say that the Beatles were the greatest rock band of all time. That is bullshit. They were a bunch of British pussies with no actual life behind their music. But the Eagles? They are part of America. Their sound is so real. Listen to Joe Walsh. Glenn Frey. These men can sing! This is the music that somebody hears when they are driving down a road in New Mexico with tumbleweed and nothing but stars in the sky. Do you hear the drummer? That is Don Henley! He is a magician. If you learn to play the drums like this guy, you can own the world."

Kirk thought of these things. He remembered the best of his father. When he needed to quiet his mind, he swallowed an oxy and played the music of his childhood on Spotify. It was always the Eagles that he listened to.

# Oliver

Oliver got a phone call from his doctor one afternoon, while sitting in his patrol car, waiting to pull over reckless drivers. The state trooper had gotten a routine physical just one week earlier. Oliver was a healthy guy and had gotten the physical to beef up his life insurance policy for Talulah and the one son they had together. Oliver loved being a father and his life felt fuller than ever before. The doctor asked Oliver to come back to the office tomorrow. He had found something "amiss" in Oliver's bloodwork.

The next day, Oliver sat in the doctor's waiting room and read a pamphlet about "Signs of a Heart Attack". He was unconcerned, as he had no blood pressure problems and there was no history of it in his family. He looked around at the other patients who sat in upholstered chairs, which were made to look plush and inviting, while being utilitarian at the same time. There was an elderly couple who were watching the news, a middle-aged couple in the middle of a spat and a malodorous hipster who reeked of marijuana. Oliver glanced at his watch. He needed to get out of here and head to a soccer game for his son.

A young woman in hot pink scrubs brought him back to a treatment room. "The doctor will be right with you," she assured with a smile. Thankfully, the doctor entered merely 90 seconds after the young woman left. He wore reading glasses and looked at his computer as he spoke to Oliver.

"In looking at your bloodwork, I found that you have an elevated PSA," the doctor stated in a monotone voice. "This is the Prostate Specific Antigen. It can be an indicator of prostate cancer. Ordinarily, I would not be concerned about this number in someone your age. However, you stated in your history that your father has had prostate cancer. This predisposes you to getting it, because it is a very genetic disease. Furthermore, men of African-American descent have a much higher risk of getting prostate cancer."

Oliver felt numb. It was as though this doctor was talking in space, where sound does not travel. The MD kept talking and booked a prostate biopsy for Oliver on the following week. Oliver took the business card on which the appointment time was scheduled from the young woman in scrubs. He got into his GMC truck and drove to his son's soccer game. He would never remember much from that afternoon. It was completely blank, a smear of amnesia in a guy who was otherwise a watchful warrior to all who knew him.

It was not until Oliver got home with his son and looked at Talulah that he realized what was happening. He had an uncharacteristic and furious meltdown in the back shed. Talulah stayed near him, looking afraid and intermittently peeking out the door to make sure their son had not gone into the back yard to hear his father scream for the first time.

*"Fucking prostate cancer!? That asshole brought out the fucking battering ram, when it might not even BE cancer! He doesn't know what the fuck he is talking about! I don't have fucking cancer! How dare he say that to me!? Oh, and Talulah, listen to this! He called me an 'African-American'! My mother is Jamaican! We are not Africans!"*

Oliver did not sleep for the entire week until the biopsy. His wife tried everything to console him, she gave him spare Xanax pills that she saved for air travel, she plied him with offers of blowjobs and made his favorite food for dinner. But nothing worked, and nothing would, until Oliver was certain that the biopsy was negative for cancer.

That moment never came, because the biopsy revealed the presence of cancer cells in Oliver's prostate. The doctor was relatively respectful when he broke the news to Oliver. He was not reading verbatim from his computer that day. He simply stated that Oliver had the option of radiation to the prostate to eradicate the cancer cells or he could have his entire prostate removed surgically. Oliver was proud of himself for not ripping the doctor's framed diploma from the University of Mississippi off the taupe walls of the office and smashing the glass all over the carpeting.

Immediately after this appointment, Oliver drove to his Dad's house at 4 pm. They sat out back and drank bourbon. Oliver had wanted to hunt, to find and kill whatever he could, but his father forbade it. "This is not a time for shooting, Ollie. Your head is a mess. And I would know, because I had prostate cancer too." Oliver's father did not say that he had a full life despite the cancer, although he did have to wear pads for urinary leakage. But he *could* still get it up at least once a week. He did not say this to his son because men are men, and there are some things they don't say out loud.

The two men sat outside and drank until the sun came up the next morning. Oliver knew that he could not go to work. He was tired in a way that he had never known before. He crawled into the twin bed of his childhood and slept like the dead, as his Jamaican mother cooked with the kind of worry that only a mother whose child has been diagnosed with illness knows.

# Tom

Tom had begun the injection process for his pain. He flew to the Newark Liberty International Airport every week to see Dr. Shah. Dr. Shah numbed the area first and then did a series of needle pricks around his patient's tailbone and the spot between the anus and the testicles. While Tom had not noticed enormous improvement yet, he felt like less of fraud with his wife Casey, as she now understood what he was going through. Tom also decreased his hours at work. He was unable to explain to the editor of the wine magazine why he could not fly as often, but Dr. Shah wrote a letter of medical necessity which Tom presented to his employer, and it said nothing about rectal spasms or erectile dysfunction.

Tom found a Pelvic Floor Physical Therapist, just as Dr. Shah had suggested. She worked out of a small office in Providence. Her name was Sally and she was British. Just as all other things surrounding his diagnosis, Tom had no idea what to expect when he went to his first appointment of physical therapy.

Tom was the only person in her waiting room. Sally came into the waiting room to introduce herself. She wore a white lab coat, and she personally brought Tom into a private treatment room. She was extremely well-spoken, professional and archly devoted to her chosen line of work. This woman showed Tom a plastic three-dimensional model of the male pelvis.

She began by showing him the muscles of the pelvic floor. "These muscles must expand and retract, based on the bodily functions necessary at any given moment," she informed him, her face like a patient teacher's. "For instance, when you go to the loo for a pee or BM, these little muscles must widen and lengthen so you can void properly. Then, when you are finished, the muscles will shorten and return to where they were at rest. We are all holding in gas and urine right now, without even thinking about it. It's remarkable, isn't it?"

Sally ran her long, tapered fingers along the muscles on the plastic model as she spoke. "These are the saddle muscles," she explained. "They would be in contact with a horse when riding. They span from the front of the pubic bone, where the penis attaches, and they extend all the way back to the rectum. The tricky part of treating fellows like you is that these muscles are so tight that they do not allow men to have sex or use the loo without pain. My job is to stretch them. And then for you to learn how to relax them yourself."

"How can they be stretched?" Tom asked. Twenty minutes later, after much discussion and encouragement, Sally talked Tom into placing her gloved finger into his rectum. Only Sally called the rectum the 'back passage'. *A nice turn of phrase,* Tom thought. *Leave it to the Brits to call the asshole something elegant.*

"This is the most effective way to stretch out the muscles," Sally explained, as Tom lay in the fetal position and his practitioner sat in a chair behind him. He had winced when her lubricated finger first entered his anus, but then Tom began noticing that he was relaxing around this odd presence in his pelvic cavity. Sally found spots within his rectum, strange areas of muscular twitching, that subsided after her finger remained there long enough. She told Tom to breathe through his nose and send air into his belly. When she was finished, Sally left the room and told Tom to change back into his clothing and sit in a chair.

As he pulled up his pants and fastened his belt, Tom felt sore. But he also felt an opening within his testicles and penis, one he had not felt in a while. Sally returned to the treatment room with her plastic model of the male pelvis. She gesticulated as she talked. Her enthusiasm was infectious. "Now you might be able to realize that when we stretch the pelvis through the back passage, you will start to feel a lengthening of your muscles. In time, this will allow you to go to the loo and have successful arousal and ejaculation with more ease."

Tom was dumbfounded. This physical therapist had spoken about his most shameful problems with utter detachment, she had made his treatment seem as natural as taking care of a torn rotator cuff or tennis elbow. "Here's what we will do in the future," Sally delineated. "You should come here once a week. We will continue the internal stretches of the back passage, but you must also incorporate yoga stretches and meditation into your lifestyle, for this to have lasting results. The more you invest in your recovery, the faster you will return to having satisfactory relations with your wife. Which I think you will agree with me is every man's primary concern."

Tom returned home that night feeling as though he was newly accepted to culinary school once more. He had stopped at a green grocer's and butcher to select excellent ingredients for dinner. He prepared a wonderful meal for Casey and the girls, with the skill and elan he had forgotten he had mastered years back. While getting into bed, Tom noticed the stirrings of a hard-on. Casey was already asleep, and he did not want to tempt fate by racing back into the game. Instead, he got into the shower and rubbed one out silently in the hot stream of water, though the pleasure of his first orgasm in months made him want to shout from the rooftops.

# Rick

It has been a full year since Rick began his treatment with Dr. Ashtiju. He has dropped over fifty pounds, works out regularly and is able to masturbate four times a week with full release. His main problem is what to do about finding an outlet for his new sex drive. He has tried going into the master bedroom and bringing meals on trays to his wife Nicole. While Nicole eats the sandwiches and soups that her husband prepares, she pulls away when Rick attempts to kiss her cheek or hold her hand.

Rick is torn about what to do regarding his marriage. While he loves his wife and was raised to be faithful, he feels it would be a waste to not be able to get laid again. Especially after his hard-won journey to be able to have any drive whatsoever. He isn't proud of what he does next. Rick knows that he cannot go to a local tavern and meet a woman. Everyone in town knows him and Pittsburgh is a small city. Instead, he logs onto a website and finds single women who also want an anonymous screw.

The first time he does this, he meets a woman around his age in a local motel. Rick is embarrassed when he pays for the room and sees that they offer a "short stay". The place is seedy, and he checks to make sure his work truck is parked away from the street, so no one would see his license plate. The woman knocks on the door where Rick is waiting. The lights are dim, and he cannot see her fully, though he guesses her to be around fiftyish. *Maybe she is in an unhappy marriage, like mine,* he muses.

This woman does not want to talk. Instead, she hikes up her skirt and bends over the King-sized motel bed. Rick unzips his blue jeans, uses his teeth to open a condom and fucks her quickly. There are mirrors on the walls, and Rick can barely see the woman's face behind her long curtain of hair. When he finishes, which does not take long, he wants to look at this woman and talk to her. But he does not have the chance, because she has already pulled down her skirt and is cleaning herself in the bathroom.

This is the beginning of a series of one-night screws, each of them at the same motel, and all of them with total strangers who Rick would never see again. The sex is different with each of the women. Some of them are screamers who like to ride him and beg him to tweak their nipples. Others want to be spanked and fucked hard with legs spread on the dresser. Some of them want to suck his dick and swallow his ejaculate.

While Rick looks forward to his random encounters with these women and finds each one exciting and unique, he begins to see that there is a sameness to what he is up to. The motel room is always seedy and disgusting, the women are always aloof and after their own pleasure, and there is absolutely no connection he feels between himself and each of the pussies he is pounding. Rick knows that he is living every man's fantasy. There will likely never be a moment of reckoning where one of these women would contact his wife. Rick suspects that these women have more to lose than Rick does, with their wild and desperate longing for aberrant sex. They probably have professions, children and partners who they are trying to protect.

And this is the niggling part of the whole she-bang for Rick. These women that he meets have partners who might actually be upset if they discovered that they were cheating. But Rick does not have that with Nicole. He wonders if she might simply feel relieved to discover that he is getting his rocks off and is no longer a bother to her. Rick finds it difficult to fall asleep at night again. He stops bringing trays of food down to Nicole. Because what he cannot bear is the cold wall of disgust that she has built up against him. It is that disgust that brings him back to the motel, week after week. Even if these strangers do not want to talk to him or be taken on an actual date, at least they do not shudder at his touch. No, they welcome it. Rick would take 17 minutes of connection over a lifetime of detachment.

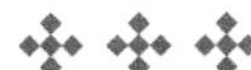

# Sheila

Sheila's medical practice was thriving. She was booked for months into the future and found herself being very satisfied on her drive home from work each day. She considered buying a home in Pittsburgh. She has not yet discussed this with Stacy, as this is a very huge step towards commitment. While Sheila and Stacy moved to Pittsburgh together, which was a risk, they had never really discussed making their relationship more permanent than it was right now.

Not only was Sheila's professional life blossoming, but her sex drive had returned in a way that she was stunned to greet. Stacy and Sheila had sex several nights during the week. And it wasn't just Stacy initiating it, either. Sheila began meeting Stacy's friends for cocktails in the evenings and was expanding her social circle. The two women were "out" as far as being lesbians. While this felt unusual to Sheila, to be able to declare her sexual proclivities in public, she loved being able to stroke Stacy's thigh over dinner in public.

It was at this high point in Sheila's life when she heard the news of her father's illness. Farrokh had called his only daughter to tell her that his kidneys were failing. "They want me to go to hemodialysis, Sheila," he explained. "I find that treatment to be disgusting. Have you ever seen people hooked up to the tubes? I refuse to do this!" Farrokh declared. Sheila was fully aware of what her father's diagnosis meant. She had been trained as a urologist, after all, and understood the delicate role that the kidneys played in stripping toxins from the bloodstream. If the kidneys were no longer working, then hemodialysis was the only treatment available to filter the blood and allow a person to keep on living.

Sheila did not like the thought of her father on hemodialysis. It was a tough way to live and patients undergoing such treatment were forced to go for treatments three times weekly, for hours at a time, often for the rest of their lives. They reported profound fatigue, they could not travel anywhere because they had to be close to a treatment center, and their bodies did not always take well to this artificial "blood cleaning" that they had to endure. Yet the only alternative to hemodialysis was death.

Sheila tried to talk sense into her father. "Dad, hemodialysis is not so bad. You can still have a good life. I have treated patients who have been on dialysis for over a decade. It will prolong your life significantly. You cannot give up right away." But Farrokh was adamant. "I am not going to live this way! It isn't your body, it is mine!" Sheila's hands shook as she held her cell phone close to her face. There she was once again, though miles away, up in front of the man who had done everything to judge and control the outcome of her life. After all these years, her father still held the power to buckle the knees of this prominent physician.

The doctor knew the outcome of patients who refused hemodialysis. They usually had about 7-10 days to live. It was a painful death, as the toxins in the body built within it, the limbs became swollen and edematous, the body emitted the foulest of odors during the last hours of life. Sheila could not say any of this to her father. Instead, she told him that she would get in her car, drive to Houston and be near him. Farrokh was strangely silent then; it was his tacit consent. He had never been quiet before, so Sheila knew she had to act quickly before he could refuse.

As Sheila pulled out her suitcase and began madly shoving her summertime clothing into it, Stacy arrived back home and reached for her lover's hand to ask her what was happening. Sheila sat on their bed, head hung, and told her lover that she would be leaving for Houston because her father was dying. Because Stacy was also in healthcare, she understood the gravity of the situation.

Stacy's protective instinct kicked in. "You are not driving to Houston alone. You are not in the right frame of mind for that long a trip." Sheila was now quiet and unable to continue packing. "I am going with you on the drive down," Stacy commanded. "I know your family will not want to meet me. Your Muslim father would die if he knew you had a girlfriend, even though we both know he is dying anyway. I can stay in a local hotel. Nobody will know I am there. But there is no way I am letting you get down there by yourself."

Sheila and her suitcase were placed in the car by Stacy, who sat in the driver's seat. The former Texas Longhorn cheerleader drove for fifteen hours straight before stopping for a break. Stacy checked them into a hotel in Arkansas. She removed Sheila's clothing and ran hot water for the tub. Stacy sat on the floor of the hotel bathroom while Sheila lay supine and soaked.

Sheila had said nothing since the trip began. But with black-ringed eyes and a slumped spine, she looked up at her girlfriend. "*I could not have done this without you. Whatever have I done in my life to deserve finding you?*" And Sheila cried, she could have filled that tub with her tears. These were the tears of guilt for letting her father down, for living a lie as a lesbian, for feeling as though her medical degrees and accolades would never be enough. Sheila cried for hours. Stacy knelt beside her, filled the tub with more hot water and washed the doctor's back.

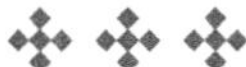

# Kirk

The band is nearing the end of their nationwide tour. They have built up a reputation as being somewhat good and have something of a following. There are a few soft openings for a record deal and the sound of the band is oozing something that feels like success. The finale of the tour is in Alaska in the summer. The guys are hyped up to spend time in The Land of the Midnight Sun. Kirk wants to write a new song about it, because he has heard that the hours of unending daylight are something quite unique.

The guys in the band are staying at a lodge-type home. There are hot Russian chicks everywhere in Alaska and they work out of drive-through coffee houses. The constant sunlight encourages lots of outdoor partying on the deck of the lodge. With the slim amount of money that the band now has to their name, they pool their resources, throw a party on the deck of the lodge and invite the hot Russians. The Russians are not aware that the band members are not all that famous, but the ruse works.

It is on this last night of the tour that Kirk's pain returns. It is searing and won't quit. Kirk is talking to a woman named Svetlana. She has cat-like eyes and a sick body. He knows that he could close the deal, that Svetlana would very quickly remove her clothing and do whatever he wants. But the pain in his penis and testicles is so awful that he tries to keep talking and keeping Svetlana interested while he drinks half a bottle of Jack Daniels.

Kirk and Svetlana are finally alone on the deck. All the other band members are fucking in separate rooms. Kirk excuses himself to go into his bedroom. The pain is building, it is scorching, and his rectum feels like there is a hot poker in it. Kirk takes four pills of oxy, smashes them with a tin in which he carries his weed, and snorts the small white particles. He then goes back to the deck to get Svetlana. The rest of the night is a blur. When he awakens, the Russians are gone, and Kirk hears the guys in the band packing their things to leave.

The guys fly from Anchorage to Seattle and then begin their long drive home, back to New York City. The excitement of the tour is fading, and the guys know that they need to return to some semblance of reality. They might have to get jobs as bartenders or Uber drivers. No one will look at them like the Russian women did. They will just be regular guys now, with regular lives. Well, the other guys in the band would be. Kirk is slowly realizing that his pelvic pain is not going to just disappear. It has found a way into his life, an insidious way of taking away his manhood.

Kirk feels a sense of profound isolation. There is a not a single person with whom he can talk to about his problem. The bigger problem is that vocalizing this pain might then make it real. It might give the pain even more of an identity and Kirk cannot fathom how much more this dark pain will take from his life. How much more could it? If all the drinking and drugs could not push it away, how would Kirk learn to live with this problem?

The days on the tour bus back to New York bled into a wash of misery. The pain, the depression caused by the pain, and the starkly bleak future is all Kirk can fixate on. It is through that pain that Kirk realizes the very thing that has shackled him all these years, even before his pelvic pain had begun. It is the memory of his father leaving. It is his Dad's drunken insistence that Kirk is going to be somebody, followed by his disappearance. It is the sound of the Eagles, of Don Henley in particular, that has become the musical score to Kirk's life. There is an Eagles song for every emotion a person could have.

For whatever reason, Kirk suddenly recalls working at the gas station with the Russian Ivan. Ivan had hired Kirk when he was underage. Ivan had a unibrow, but it always furrowed when he looked at this American teenager who was trying to pretend that he was an adult, that he was capable of taking care of himself, and that it did not matter to Kirk that his father was gone. Ivan had always known that this had mattered, Kirk realizes on that bus. Ivan had gone to Kirk's high school graduation, he had stood like a large, protective Papa Bear in the bleachers and had thrust $300 of cash into Kirk's hand afterwards. "I vant you to do somezing good with your life," the Russian had said. It had taken every ounce of dickishness to prevent Kirk from crying in that moment. Kirk had barely thanked the Russian, turned on his heel and followed his friends to a drinking party.

Through the shaking withdrawals from his oxycodone, Kirk is at last able to see that his Dad's dream for his son has ended terribly. That the stardom of being the drummer in a band has come with a terrible price and that Kirk has not followed Ivan's advice of doing "somezing" good with his life. Kirk feels something open in his chest, a peeling away of the lining of his heart and he wonders if maybe, just maybe, he can turn his life around.

# Oliver

Oliver's urologist was far better than his primary physician. He was a straight shooter. This specialist had been the man who performed the prostate biopsy. The doctor had recommended sedation for the procedure: "Most men find it less stressful to not be awake during the biopsy, as it can be unsettling." Oliver had declined the sedation, because he wanted to be in control over his body. This had been a terrible mistake, Oliver learned, because the biopsy involved having a hollow needle shoved up his rectum while it took small pieces of tissue from several parts of his prostate gland. It was not only painful as the device grabbed samples of tissue from several portions of his prostate, but it sounded like the jolt of a staple gun each time the tissue was retrieved.

Having unnecessarily endured the biopsy while being perfectly alert and coherent, Oliver grew to trust his urologist. He appreciated how the physician spoke to him, in a no-bullshit kind of way. "Your prostate cancer is somewhat aggressive, so I am very glad that we caught it when we did," The urologist said. "If left untreated, this type of cancer would have spread into your bladder and surrounding bones of the pelvis. But if we remove the prostate from your body, we can stop that from happening."

This information was a lot for Oliver to take in. He didn't want his prostate removed. Oliver's Dad had been treated with the radioactive seeds. This seemed like a less drastic approach. Oliver asked his urologist, "Couldn't I get some form of radiation instead? I have read online that this is another way to target the cancer and I would be able to keep my prostate."

The doctor's reply, though not exactly what Oliver wanted to hear, was right to the point. "I have seen a lot of cases of prostate cancer. And I have been treating this disease for two decades now. If you were in your sixties, as I assume your father is, I would be more than happy to treat this with radiation. But given your young age and how aggressive this cancer appears to be, the radiation may not get all of the cancer cells. It will also burn the surrounding tissues and prevent future surgery in this area of your body, should you ever need it. If I was in your shoes, I would get a prostatectomy, or prostate removal."

*Could things get any worse?* Oliver wondered. *What kind of a life will I have if the doctor removed my entire prostate?* The doctor seemed to read Oliver's mind in that moment. "If we remove your prostate, you may have an almost full return of your sexual life. It won't happen right away. But with the advances we have made in surgery, I can spare the nerves that control a good erection. You won't have any liquid when you ejaculate without a prostate. But you will have the same sensation of a climax. You should also expect some degree of urinary leakage after the surgery. This often resolves after a few months."

Oliver drove home, his mind clouded and boggy. He could barely listen to the urologist's talk about the side-effects of having his prostate removed, because his foremost concern was ridding his body of this "aggressive" cancer. While he was furious about the entire ordeal, he felt a little better upon talking to his urologist and was not tempted to tear the guy's diploma from medical school off the wall. Oliver's fate rested in the hands of a skilled surgeon and Oliver trusted this man. That was important.

That same evening, Oliver and Talulah stayed up half the night together. Talulah spoke of wanting another child and Oliver wanted nothing more than to give her this. But that option was no longer on the table. Once his prostate came out, he would not be able to sire any future children. Oliver told Talulah that he might piss himself and need pads or diapers for a while; or maybe forever. Talulah took his hand. *I don't care about that,* her eyes said. But the thing that Oliver could not bring himself to say out loud was about the cancer itself. Why had these cells chosen his prostate to embed themselves within? Other people got cancer every day. But not a soldier from the Army, not a state trooper, not a guy who had married a great girl, just as their lives were essentially beginning.

Oliver made up his mind. He decided to undergo a prostatectomy, otherwise known as removal of the prostate. He trusted his doctor and felt in his gut that this was the right path to follow. Talulah drove him to the hospital on the day of the surgery and held his hand the entire way. Oliver was terrified, despite the confidence he held in his decision. As the liquid anesthesia entered his left brachial vein, Oliver saw the faces of all the men he had killed as a sniper. He had never seen those targets that he excelled at hitting as being actual *people*. Not until now. As Oliver's breathing slowed and a tube was pushed into his trachea, this sea of Iraqi and Afghani people was somehow returning to Oliver's line of vision, as if a karmic sword was cutting though his life, taking away his prostate for all that he had done in the name of war.

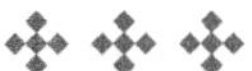

# Tom

While Tom's pelvic pain had been improving with his injections and the help of his British physical therapist Sally, he was dispirited by the fact that his symptoms would often return out of nowhere, even when Tom was doing everything that he was told by the medical community. There were weeks of almost pain-free living, but they were invariably followed by return of the rectal spasms and discomfort in Tom's penis. It seemed grossly unfair that Tom had found the best of professionals to help him and had curtailed his wine drinking by eighty percent, only to still have these symptoms.

There was some improvement though, he had to admit. Tom could now endure lengthy plane rides. He attributed this to a few factors. First, Tom meditated for up to an hour in the chapels of each airport before he boarded a plane. The silence within these chapels and the sense of people with multiple faiths and even more problems filled Tom with a sense of peace. Secondly, Sally had told Tom to use a cushion on the plane, at a desk or in his car. This specialty cushion had a cutout of the saddle region, which prevented Tom's pelvic floor muscles from getting compressed in sitting. Thirdly, Dr. Nathan Shah had recommended application of cannabis oil to Tom's rectum to treat the spasms. The combination of these interventions was helping Tom resume his normal life once more. Finally, Tom's constipation was not nearly as bothersome, he had made dietary changes, drank more water and was even educated by Sally the physical therapist on "the mechanics of defecation".

"You have got to be kidding me!" Tom teased Sally, when she brought up this topic. "Since when do physical therapists know anything about how to crap?" Sally was pleased to be able to talk about this matter. She pulled out the plastic pelvic model and touched the anal sphincter with reverence. "I must tell you how powerful it is to be able to help people to poo in the most natural way possible," she replied, in her English accent. "Many people struggle with constipation, but especially those with tight pelvic floor muscles, like you. Having regular bowel movements makes all the difference in one's quality of life."

Tom had to agree with Sally on this point. Since he was able to have daily BM's, Tom found that he had a lot less tension in his perineum. This also had a spill-over effect onto his sex life and ability to get hard and stay hard until he came. Tom was able to achieve semi-arousal when out with his wife Casey, at a bar, restaurant, wherever. This had not been possible for him in years. When the couple arrived back at home, Casey would often ask Tom how she would best be able to please him. Sometimes, it was manual sex, and she needed to avoid the tip of his penis, so as to not elicit pain. Other times, she would stroke his testicles while he grew harder, and he would give her oral sex simultaneously. There were nights when Tom could penetrate his wife and they could go at it for up to thirty minutes. While things were not as they were before his Chronic Pelvic Pain Syndrome had begun, Tom and Casey were able to have sex again. Casey was thrilled, but Tom was still disenchanted by the lack of full return of sexual function.

Things were better than they had been before he started treatment, Tom realized. But when would he be able to stop this treatment? When could he have his life back, without all these appointments with doctors, his physical therapist and needing to set aside countless hours for meditation?

On a particularly frustrating day, when the weather of Providence was cold and raw, Tom asked Sally if he might be able to cut back on treatment sessions. "Well, we could decrease the frequency that you come to see me. Instead of coming here once a week, you could cut back to twice a month and see how your symptoms fare." Tom followed Sally's instructions but was angry to realize that his pelvic pain came roaring back without his weekly physical therapy appointments. With all his reading on the subject, Tom knew that Chronic Pelvic Pain Syndrome was indeed, chronic. It would likely never go away completely, but the requirement of seeing specialists indefinitely was time-consuming and very irksome.

Sally understood Tom's frustration as no one else in his life could. Perhaps it was because she treated this condition all day long, but also it may have been because of her strange devotion to the muscles of the "back passage". Whatever the reason, Sally was Tom's safe harbor. She was the keeper of his secrets and held them as carefully as though they were written on slips of paper, stacked up neatly in a locked cupboard. Sally knew about Tom's previous drinking to hide his symptoms. She knew that his wife Casey had suspected that he was cheating on her, because of his lack of interest in sex. Sally also knew that when Tom's teenaged girls were acting up and he had no patience for their chatter or shopping habits.

Sally sat in front of Tom and told him how to handle the next step in his recovery. "You could try stretching your own pack passage with your fingers. You would be performing self-treatment to lengthen the muscles of the pelvic floor. The effect is very similar to what I am doing here." *As bizarre as it was having Sally's index finger in Tom's ass, he found it even more weird to imagine doing this himself.*

Sally picked up on the dubious look on Tom's face. "Alternatively, you could have your wife Casey come into the office and learn how to do what I do. This works well for many couples. She could perform these stretches and you would have more lasting results and fewer painful episodes." *Which is worse?* Tom thought. *Doing this myself or having Casey do this to me? She has been through enough. She stayed by me in the worst years of my condition. I cannot possibly ask this of her.*

Instead, Tom kept his once weekly appointments with Sally. He figured it was worth the time spent there to prevent the return of the horrendous pain he had once known. The date of Tom and Casey's twentieth wedding anniversary was fast approaching. He wanted to take her someplace very meaningful. He had seen wineries all over the world. But where would he take the most important person in his life?

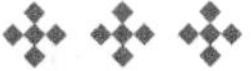

# Rick

Rick eventually stopped going to the motels to meet random women. This happened because his son Francis was home from college for the summer and Rick felt too guilty cheating on the kid's mother. Even though Francis was out with his own friends most evenings, Rick couldn't bear the thought of bumping into his son in the kitchen at midnight while reeking of sex. But things were no better between Rick and his wife Nicole. They were like roommates who lived in opposite ends of the house. These days, they barely spoke at all.

There came a day when Rick returned to see Dr. Sheila Ashtiju. He needed to come clean about his philandering, and she was just the person to tell. This doctor was like a priestess without the white collar or religious judgement. Rick was also able to tell her that he was doing better with his erections and was getting them consistently in the morning again. He had proven that he was able to reach a climax successfully, but that was with the strangers in the short stay motel. These days, he was back to masturbating, as his wife was still ignoring him.

Not only was Dr. Ashtiju unfazed by the random sexual encounters that Rick described, she seemed pleased with his progress from a medical perspective. "That is really good news, Rick," Dr. Ashtiju replied. "By coming here, you have addressed 50% of the problem of erectile dysfunction. I am not sure you need to keep coming back anymore."

Rick was startled. "What do you mean, I don't have to come back?" Rick replied. "You just said I have only addressed 50% of the problem?"

Dr. Ashtiju looked him squarely in the eye. "The other 50% of your erectile dysfunction is due to your marriage to a partner with whom you are not connected." The doctor paused for several seconds. She knew what she was doing. "Have you ever asked yourself if you could have a satisfying relationship with someone else? Have you ever given yourself permission to be happy?" Rick was shocked. The possibility of leaving Nicole had never crossed his mind.

It took him about two months, during which he spent time with Francis, before his kid went back to college and the Steelers were back on the television. There was something about the crispness of that fall air that stirred something inside Rick. He walked into his wife's bedroom and told her he would be filing for a divorce. Rick would give Nicole the house and he would keep the plumbing business. Nicole said very little, both then and in the judge's chambers when the divorce was finalized.

Immediately thereafter, Rick was not yet ready to begin dating. He still missed Nicole, despite the years without sex, or even talking, for that matter. He got an apartment in Washington Heights and spent time with friends. These were guy friends, who also admitted to having very little sex or communication in their marriages. He bought season tickets to the Steelers and flew to other cities to watch them play. He stopped going to the office of Dr. Ashtiju but would occasionally run into her at Heinz Field. This was because the doctor hung out with another woman and *they* also had season tickets to the Steelers. Rick wasn't sure what surprised him more:

that the doctor liked the NFL or that she was a lesbian! Rick was baffled to discover that a lesbian could have understood his male sexual problems so well.

Rick was not looking to get remarried. He was not even sure he wanted to live with a woman again. He was driving to a job out near Butler, in the hills on the outskirts of the city, where he saw a sign outside a home that read "Pups for Sale". He entered the home and inquired about the dogs. A tiny French bulldog was placed on his lap. He paid cash for the baby, named her Lola and took her home. Lola and Rick were instantly best friends. Rick fell asleep at night to the sound of his dog snoring. He awoke each morning and felt alive again. He had a new motto in life. *If you want sex, get a woman. If you want true love, get a dog.*

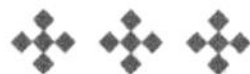

# Kirk

Kirk returned home after the music tour. He did not get another apartment with the guys from the band and he moved back in with his mother. It was an awkward situation, living in the same place that still smelled of his father's Camel cigarettes from over a decade after he had vanished. Kirk's mother now had a new boyfriend, but this guy was a quiet workaholic and Kirk had little contact with him. Kirk went to the gas station in Garfield to look for Ivan the Russian. Ivan immediately hugged the young man and slapped him on the back. "I vas afraid I vould never see you again!" Ivan shouted. The Russian bear of a man re-offered Kirk a job pumping gasoline. But that wasn't all that Ivan offered Kirk.

Ivan somehow sensed the depth of Kirk's addiction to painkillers. Perhaps it was the hollowness of Kirk's eyes, the skin that clung to his lanky bones, and the sores on his face which looked far worse than teenaged acne. Ivan drove Kirk to a doctor's office. The Russian had many connections, but one of them was a cousin who worked as a pain management physician in Fort Lee. This doctor examined Kirk, asked him about his withdrawal symptoms, and prescribed him two months' worth of suboxone. This MD did not have a strong Russian accent, but she possessed the same 'don't fuck with me' vibe that Russians were famous for. "I am giving you a substance which should help you with your withdrawal from oxycodone.

But I am ONLY giving you a certain amount of suboxone. This is to be used as a temporary measure. Many people move from being addicted to oxy to then being addicted to suboxone. I want to be clear about this: I will not refill any more prescriptions of suboxone for you! It is your job to address your addiction and find some emotional support in a twelve-step program." Ivan was anxiously pacing the waiting room when Kirk exited the doctor's office.

Kirk joined a local Narcotics Anonymous group and went to nightly meetings. The suboxone prescribed by the doctor did help Kirk with the symptoms of chemical dependency. It was not until Kirk stopped taking this drug that he learned how very expensive it was. The cost of suboxone was $800 per month. It had been Ivan who had paid for both the doctor's visit and the cost of the medication. Kirk sheepishly showed up for work at the gas station after discovering this. But Ivan would hear no thank yous, no attempts to pay back any of the money.

Kirk continued to have symptoms of Chronic Pelvic Pain Syndrome. Luckily, there was an online support group for that, too. Kirk was surprised to find a large group of guys who had exactly the same groin problems that he did. It was this sense of support, all coming from a satellite in the sky, that allowed Kirk to manage the terrible problems which had led to his drug addiction in the first place. During the very cold winter months when Kirk worked outside pumping gas, he would occasionally pee himself. While he was mystified as to why this would be, it was only after posing this question to his online support group that he got an answer. The reason that he was pissing himself when the weather got cold was that his groin muscles were squeezing so tightly to brace against the frigid temperatures, causing urine to escape his urethra. Not only was Kirk learning about the anatomy of his problem, but he was learning ways to fix it. One guy in the group suggested that Kirk purchase one of those disposable temporary hot packs that skiers use to keep their hands warm, and to place the hot pack in the crotch of his boxer briefs when the weather went below a certain temperature. Kirk did exactly that and was happy to find that the hot pack stopped the peeing by keeping his groin muscles warm.

Even though Kirk was clean and sober, and his pelvic symptoms were somewhat better than they had been, there were still some very dark days. Kirk had once been on a path to be a star, and now he was a gas attendant. He had few friends and could not go out to bars to find chicks and get laid. Kirk was not drumming very often, because his drug recovery had to take first place in his life. While it felt good to no longer need drugs to get him through the day, the physical pain of his condition and the emotional pain of his past were often more than he could bear.

Ivan invited Kirk over to his family's house for dinners every Saturday night. The Russian had a chubby wife and two young children. There was food aplenty on the table and Kirk knew that Ivan was abstaining from his chilled vodka with the meal out of respect for his friend. The smells of the food, the rough housing of the children and the protective presence of the Russian bear reminded Kirk of a certain song from the Eagles. This was the first time that Kirk had ever thought of this particular song as having any relevance to his life, and yet he heard it, as clear as anything. The song was "Desperado".

Kirk looked across the table at his 'father' Ivan. Their eyes met and the Russian bear lifted his chin in what was unmistakably deep pride.

# Tom

The Douro River runs westbound through the Iberian Peninsula. It begins in Spain and snakes through the countryside of Portugal before opening its mouth into the Atlantic Ocean. The land along the Douro River is quite steep and these hills create the fertile valley through which the river runs. This land is still sparsely inhabited, with the exception of farmers who herd sheep and cultivate olives and grapes. The soil in this region of the world is full of shale. It was very well suited to the type of grapes used to make port wine.

Tom had decided upon the Douro Valley as the place to bring his wife Casey for their twentieth wedding anniversary. There was a boat trip to take them down the Douro River, so she could witness the rows of grapes flanking the grand water passage. While Tom had been on this tour a few times, the sight of the elegant rows of grapes stacked up along the countryside was something which never failed to amaze him.

During his treatment in pelvic floor physical therapy in Rhode Island, Tom had finally found the courage to ask his wife if she would be interested in learning the techniques that Sally employed to stretch out his rectum. Casey immediately replied that she would not mind learning any technique that could help heal her husband from pelvic pain. So, Casey came to his very next physical therapy session. Sally performed the inter-rectal stretching on Tom, followed by Casey. All the while,

Sally asked Tom if Casey was using the same amount of pressure and getting to the same places internally that Sally was able to reach. Casey was a fast learner and now performed this technique with Tom three times weekly. It actually brought the couple very close together and improved arousal and climax for the sex that ensued after the rectal release.

Tom watched Casey's face light up as they boarded the small river boat in Portugal. The boat stopped at a few of the vineyards and gave the travelers, there were about a dozen of them, a chance to taste some of the local port. There was one lovely vineyard in particular that stood out amongst the others. The owner's name was Rui and after showing the tour group what was the harvesting of the grapes in the cool air of the valley, he brought them into a farmhouse with large windows and roughhewn wooden tables with benches. The group sat down in this old stone building and drank three different types of port. They ate freshly made bread and dipped it in deep green olive oil. They savored bits of chocolate and salted almonds.

Rui spoke through much of the tasting, guiding the travelers in what to expect from the various kinds of port. "This vineyard has been in my family for ten generations. We are very proud to maintain this land to be able to keep growing these grapes. But this is not an easy business. I will give you a history lesson to help you understand." Casey was spell-bound. She was sipping Lagrima, a white port which translated into the word for a "tear", due to the robust droplet the port made as it slid down the side of a glass.

Rui continued to talk to the room. "It was in the mid 1800's that a small bug came to find these gorgeous fields. It was called Phyllox. This little bug infected and wiped out much of our product of grapes and it did this throughout Europe.

Some say we have the Americans to blame for bringing the bug on the vines that came overseas, but I don't want to offend any Americans that may be here on vacation." Tom already knew the history of the Phyllox epidemic, but he enjoyed hearing it with Rui's accented Portuguese. And this story was now headed to the best part of all, the reason why Tom had taken Casey to this very destination. She needed to hear what happened next.

"What many people throughout Europe discovered after the Phyllox scourge was that there was a way to identify if the little bug had invaded the fields, *before it devastated the entire harvest.* Farmers learned that if they planted a rose bush at the very front of a row of planted grapes, those roses would wilt and become sick if the bug had entered the field. The farmers could then treat the Phyllox before it ruined that year's crop. In essence, the rose bush became a watchtower for the grapes. It protected the field from destruction." Casey was leaning forward on her bench, rapt with attention.

Rui continued. "Like most of Europe, it is illegal to water the grapes in the Douro Valley when the soil is dry or if we have a summer without rain. If there is a bad season, we must cut our losses and move on. But remember, we have very special soil here. It is full of shale and we cannot cultivate roses that can grow in this region of Portugal. We could try, but the roses need water, and remember, we are not allowed to water our grapes. The Portuguese are smart people. We figured out something else. We discovered that an olive tree, which grows naturally here, also possesses the ability to detect the presence of the Phyllox in our fields. Olives produce the succulent oil that you are dipping your bread into right now. So, we make money on the port and we also make money on the olives. We take great pride in our own watchtowers of the grapes. These trees stand like strong sentries to warn us when trouble is on its way. Their fruit tastes delicious as well!"

Rui was done with his history lesson. He poured extra port wine to anyone who wanted some and told the tourists their boat would be leaving in another twenty minutes. "If you drink our port as the sun sets, you will never see the world in the same way again," Rui stated with a flourish. The fading sun shone onto the grapes in the hilly fields and graced the old wooden table upon which Tom and Casey were holding their wine glasses.

Casey raised one eyebrow. "So, Tom, of all of the places in the world where you could have taken me to experience wine, why did you specifically choose this one?" Tom could have said that it was the undeniable beauty of the Douro Valley that drew him. Or that the taste of the Lagrima grapes picked thirty years ago made it his favorite dessert wine. He could have mentioned that it was inspiring to see the years of respect and pride that these individual families had taken in passing down their land as a legacy for future generations. And all of this would be true.

But the real reason that Tom had brought Casey to the Douro Valley was those olive trees. The watchtowers of the grapes. The guardians of the health of the land. Those olive trees played an essential role in the production of port wine. Without them, the grapes might have died years ago, and younger generations might not have been interested in carrying on the legacy of this particular grape. This would be a loss to society, Tom believed. Wine was his life and he honored the years of work that went into one single bottle.

Tom's life was also Casey. He honored everything that Casey had done to bring him this far. She had started a business on her own, birthed and helped to raise his daughters, and loved him when he had pushed her away. It was because of Casey that Tom had wanted to get better from his pain. She had been worth fighting for. Tom looked at his wife and found the reason in her face why he had become the watchtower for his own pain. He had stayed in one place, just like the olive tree, waiting for the signal that the pain would return. And even when it did, as he knew that it would, Tom knew that he could ward it off and that Casey would be right next to him to help. "Cheers to us, my love," he whispered, as their glasses clinked before the moon would rise over the valley.

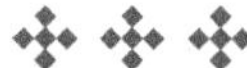

# Sheila

Sheila's father had been admitted to the same hospital in Houston where she had once worked and earned the commendation that made her a specialist in treating prostate cancer. She wore dark sunglasses and casual jeans when she returned to see him. Dr. Ashtiju did not want to be noticed by the staff who had once garnered her with praise. It had been three years since Sheila had been back to Texas. She located her father's bedroom and stopped to cross her arms and rub her own shoulders before she rounded the corner to enter it. There he was: her rock, her role model, her father, her mentor, her everything. His color was sallow, and his face and neck were swollen with fluid. As much as Sheila had seen illness and even death in her line of work, it was a whole different ball game when it was her father who was sick.

She sat at the edge of her father's hospital bed and took his hand. "I am glad that you came here," Farrokh told his daughter. "They tell me I can eat whatever I want at this point and it will not matter. I was thinking of ordering my first BLT. What do you think? Will Allah have a problem with that during my eleventh hour?" Sheila smiled through the mucous that was building in her throat. Her father had developed a sense of humor overnight. She had not been expecting this. How much morphine were the nurses giving him?

Sheila spent that entire week in the hospital. She slept in a Geri-chair next to her Dad's hospital bed and they watched ridiculous television shows together (the sort of mindless TV that Sheila had never been allowed to view as a child). Farrokh discovered that he actually liked the taste of pork products, though he couldn't eat very much. He just took small bites and smiled. Sheila knew that he was not going to last too much longer when he took ragged breaths with his mouth open, like a guppy. But she remained next to him the entire time.

It was late one evening when Sheila had drifted off into sleep in the Geri-chair that she heard her father call her name. She stood up and went to Farrokh's side. "What is it, Father?" she asked in Farsi. He was gasping for air, trying to form words with his dry, cracked lips. At last, he spoke them. These were the words that Sheila had needed her entire life. They were the words spoken when one has nothing left to hide or prove and time is running out. *"I am so proud of you. I have always known that you would not marry a man. That you are gay. I still have always loved you, my precious daughter."*

Farrokh's mouth remained open upon his death, just after he said these words. Sheila reached down to close his eyelids and jaw. She kissed his forehead and went to tell the nurse that her father was gone. The doctor then called her girlfriend Stacy, who was staying at a local hotel. "Come pick me up," Sheila said, as she looked around the main lobby of the hospital. Dr. Ashtiju knew that she would never return to this place. While it had been her beginning and a very heroic start to her professional life, Sheila no longer needed the reminder of these things for where she was headed next.

After her father's farewell admission, Sheila felt an unexpected freedom which strode alongside her deep mourning.

She went to Farrokh's memorial service and wore the requisite Prada heels. She found the shoes uncomfortable as she stood in a black suit and spoke to her relatives. When Sheila was finished putting on the show of being the perfect daughter and doctor for all to see, she slipped off her heels and called Stacy from the coat room to rescue her. Stacy pulled up to the front of the funeral home in the same Mercedes that Farrokh had bought his daughter after she graduated from medical school. Sheila leapt into the front seat. It was time to go back home to Pittsburgh.

The miles went by as the two lovers drove North. It was a long trip, but they did not want to stop and continued driving through the night. They took turns at the wheel. They talked about their years of being in the Operating Room, how they had first met and fallen in love. Sheila talked about her father. "He always seemed so invulnerable to me. That he was not really human. I was raised with that image of men and it affected me. I think that is why I like treating men with sexual dysfunction. Because I can see them as vulnerable, as people who have lost everything that means something to them. I can see men as broken and afraid. I love that I can do this." It was because of her father's death that Sheila was finally able to articulate these things which she had previously held so close.

The drive continued on the Pennsylvania Turnpike. Stacy, the ex-cheerleader of the Texas Longhorns, turned to Sheila and said, "I miss watching football. I know I am not making a lot of sense, because I have not slept in a while, but I want to go to a Steelers game. I want *US* to go to a football game together!" Sheila did not know when she nodded yes that she was agreeing to stand outside in the terrible Pittsburgh weather and watch a bunch of grown men fight over a ball.

She also did not know that she would grow to really like football and to respect the game that encompassed strategy and the gritty toil that embodied the city of Pittsburgh. And before long, Sheila and Stacy went to football games in North Face jackets and came to love the Steelers.

There was something about that drive following Farrokh's death that had changed everything. When the two women had left Houston to start over in Pittsburgh three years ago, they had never noticed the beautiful rolling hills that led up through Western Pennsylvania. They had been running away then, and people who run cannot see beauty in front of them. But now, after living together in a place so far from home and driving back, they noticed the miles of countryside, with the occasional farm to spice up the view. The greenery of the land looked like emeralds. Their eyes scanned the view, and the two women were spent of words as they neared the city of Pittsburgh. They entered the Fort Pitt Tunnel, and knew that they were almost home. Sheila was driving and felt enclosed by the tunnel, it was deep and dark and mystical. She felt her eyes flutter in exhaustion, as though she might fall asleep.

It was then that it happened. The Mercedes emerged from the tunnel. It began as a pinprick of light on the retina, and then suddenly, the city of Pittsburgh was in full panorama. The tall buildings of Downtown glittered in the distance. The sun burst through the clouds, an unusual flash of brilliance which greeted the travelers who, seconds earlier, had been wrapped in a cloak of the darkness of the tunnel. Sheila laughed, she grabbed Stacy's hand and the two of them felt the warm sun lead them home at last.

# Oliver

For several weeks after his prostate removal, Oliver had urinary leakage. He needed to wear pads and didn't want to have sex at all. Oliver's fear was that urine would leak out of his penis during sex. Yet his urologist was encouraging and said, "I am prescribing you Cialis. I want you to take it every day, even if you don't want to have sex. This will bring blood to the area and promote healing of the incisions. But you should try to have sex. The more you use your penis again, the more likely you will be to return to full erectile function."

Oliver also had pain along his abdomen. There were small scars from where the surgeon had entered his body to remove his prostate and they were smaller than bullet wounds. But they were itchy, irritating, raised little knots of tissue that formed keloids and were a pesky reminder of all that Oliver had endured to get the cancerous cells out of his body.

It turned out that the urologist was correct about a lot of things. Oliver's urinary leakage eventually stopped, and he was able to have erections which were very similar to the ones he'd had pre-surgery. His wife Talulah had been patient, understanding, and she even joined a support group for Partners of Patients with Prostate Cancer. There were a lot of men being diagnosed with this condition and it helped for their lovers to know what to expect afterwards. Every individual was different, Talulah discovered, and it was not merely the surgical or radiation procedures that took a toll on their lives.

Nobody understood the impact of a cancer diagnosis more so than the patients themselves. The biggest part of Oliver's life that changed was his reconciliation with having cancer. His rage over the diagnosis had slowly receded, like a small band of militia whose presence on the terrain of his life was too exhausted to keep fighting. Oliver recalled his past as a sniper. He thought of the men who he had killed in the Middle East, men who were younger than he was now, men who had wives and children. While Oliver knew that he had served his country and had performed his skill with excellence as a sharpshooter at that time in his life, he was now unable to carry a gun or work as a state trooper anymore. Oliver wore the fragility of life differently now. He resigned from his job with a full pension. His main focus became his wife and family.

Talulah had wanted another child before Oliver's prostate surgery. Oliver was not a man who denied his wife anything. Because Oliver's mother was Jamaican born, the couple decided to adopt an eighteen-month-old baby from that same island. Oliver and Talulah stayed in Jamaica for several weeks before they were authorized to bring their newly adopted boy home. After they arrived in an airplane back home to Alabama, Oliver's mother danced with her Jamaican grandson in the yard as she sang the songs of her homeland. Oliver and Talulah's elder son picked up sticks in the yard and fought imaginary enemies, and the two boys grew up together.

Oliver raised his two boys well. When they came of age, he took them out into the woods and taught them how to kill turkey, deer and wild boar with a crossbow. In time, the boys became as skilled with a crossbow as their father had been with a shotgun. They were often brought to the home of their grandparents, where three generations of men would prepare handmade sausages and filet venison. Oliver's Dad was thrilled to have these grandchildren around. Oliver and his father stood side by side as they manned the smoker with the meat they had harvested themselves. These two men had different skin and eye color, they looked nothing alike, but had shared the same type of cancer and had fought it, and won.

It was during those moments when Oliver grinned from ear to ear. He looked across his Dad's property and saw his mother and wife talking and laughing as they snapped off the ends of green beans for supper. In his dreams, he hovered behind his two sons and guided their hands on the crossbow, teaching them how to aim right for the head of a turkey off in the distance. This was the new imprint that remained on Oliver's brain when he fell asleep these days. He awoke each morning and said to himself, "I have everything a guy could want."

# Part II

# The Nonfiction

*"An erection is a carefully orchestrated series of events, with the central nervous system in the role of conductor."* (Goldstein, 2000)

The first segment of this book was devoted to the stories of five fictional people: four men with different pelvic problems and one female physician who treats the male pelvis. These guys represent the type of patient who seeks help from a pelvic floor physical therapist. The identities of these four guys were fabricated, but the way their lives were impacted is in keeping with how a man with pelvic difficulties perceives the world around him. I have been very fortunate to work with this population and hope that I have done a fair job honoring their stories as they get through these very unique hardships.

The second segment of the book will delve into more scientific and physiological reasons behind erectile dysfunction, pelvic pain and prostate cancer. It is compilation of research and journal articles coupled with my own experience in working with urologists, physicians, and fellow pelvic floor specialists. This part of the book is important in order to understand how each of these characters faces the challenges of pelvic floor dysfunction. It explores why pelvic pain occurs and describes the treatments that are available. These sorts of treatments are not all *widely* available, but in time and with more exposure to this specific health concern, that may change in a decade or so.

I would be remiss by not including the disclaimer that this book is not intended to diagnose, treat or cure the diagnoses listed therein. Rather, the purpose of this section is to provide information about these various pelvic problems and suggestions for how to ease the symptoms inherent with dysfunction of the male pelvis.

# Rick

Let's start by talking about the character Rick. Rick was created as a character because he has a simple medical background. He is your average, middle-aged man, carrying around a few extra pounds and finding that he no longer has the sexual response that he once did. Rick represents many men who are out there. He starts his own method of treatment by taking a testosterone supplement. This is something that many men initially start with, because A) they don't want to talk about their erectile dysfunction with anyone B) they don't want to go to a doctor, pay a copay and get prescribed a low dose of generic Viagra that may not help them and C) the testosterone marketed for the average Joe seems as safe and effective to boost virility as a vitamin shake.

In speaking with several physicians who specialize in the use of hormones, this over-the-counter use of testosterone is not that helpful for erectile dysfunction and is actually *damaging* to a man's psychological state and well-being. The first thing an MD should do if he or she suspects that their patient is low on any given hormone would be to test for it in the bloodstream. This allows the practitioner a baseline level from which to work, which then guides the MD in how much of any given hormone should be prescribed. When men begin taking testosterone supplements while not under the supervision of a physician, the effects can vary greatly. Some men may feel no change whatsoever when taking over-the-counter testos-terone, while other men very rapidly morph into Incredible Hulks, in terms of rage and erratic behavior. Furthermore, an excess of unregulated testosterone in the human body can cause heart disease, a heart attack, reduced testicular size and sleep apnea. In Rick's case, the testosterone pills he buys do not have much of an effect on his sex drive and he abandons their use after seeing Dr.Sheila Ashtiju upon his first visit. Rick's doctor tests for the hormone level in his blood and prescribes a testosterone cream to be applied to his testicles each evening. This is the mildest form of testosterone replace-ment. In actual practice, some physicians use testosterone injections or pellets, which are small capsules that are embed-ded underneath the skin to provide a long-lasting supply of the deficient hormone.

Rick responds well to his prescribed testosterone, but he also notices tremendous benefit from weight loss and regular exercise. Losing weight and engaging in physical activity both aid in increasing blood flow into the pelvis and enhance spon-taneous erections. Does everyone remember Jack LaLanne? For those of you born after 1984, Jack LaLanne was a fitness and nutritional guru, as well as being a motivational speaker for health. Mr. LaLanne once gave an interview wherein he stated, "I wake up every morning with an erection a cat can't scratch." Jack lived until he was 96 years old and continued to brag about his sexual prowess until late in his life, thus proving the link between exercise and a satisfactory sexual re-sponse. Many men with typical erectile dysfunction may find an improvement in symptoms by adding cardio activity, light weight training and dietary modifications, like limiting alcohol consumption, into their lives.

Now let's go back to the dreaded questionnaire that Rick fills out for Dr. Sheila Ashtiju before he meets her in the treatment room. The first part of the questionnaire asks very specific sexual questions. One of the most noteworthy questions from a health-care provider's viewpoint when looking at sexual function, is this: "Are you able to get an erection sufficient enough for penetrative sex? Are you then able to maintain that erection to continue with sex until climax?" In Rick's case, he didn't need to respond to that question, because we as the readers already know that he has not had sex with his wife Nicole in quite some time. But we also know that Rick cannot get an erection necessary for basic masturbation. He is not responding to manual sex, and therefore has almost no erectile function whatsoever.

Then there is the second part of the questionnaire wherein Dr. Ashtiju asks Rick if he is living through any major life stressors, like divorce, bankruptcy, death of a loved one, or raising problem children. Rick is completely miffed by this line of questioning; he is even somewhat offended by being asked these personal questions that appear to have no link to his sex life. We as the readers are allowed a glimpse into how this physician is treating her patient. Dr. Sheila Ashtiju is trying to find a connection between a stressful life event and the onset of Rick's erectile dysfunction. It isn't until Rick thinks about this that he realizes that the timeframe of when his erectile dysfunction first manifested itself was when his wife Nicole stopped taking care of herself. It isn't simply that Nicole didn't want to have sex; no, Nicole is undergoing a major depressive episode that renders her unable to be a wife, mother or someone who can leave the house to work at the plumbing business. Rick is now thrust into the role of the primary caregiver for the entire household.

What does that level of stress do to the body? More specifically, what does it do to a man's sex drive, and why? The arc of Rick's story is characteristic of sexual dysfunction, because of the body's interplay of communication between the adrenal glands and hormone production. The adrenal glands sit on top of the kidneys. They produce the chemical cortisol, which is the body's main stress hormone. This is the "fight or flight" hormone and it allows the body to respond to high levels of stress for short periods of time. When the body is under duress for long periods of time, however, too much cortisol is released, and the adrenal glands become depleted of their bank of stored cortisol. The diagnosis that occurs when a person has been running on empty for far too long is known as "adrenal fatigue".

People in adrenal fatigue often have a very low sex drive. But why? This is because small amounts of cortisol are the building blocks of testosterone. Without any cortisol, the body cannot produce its own testosterone, and the urge for sex becomes diminished. Rick's dip in arousal and the ability to get an erection happened just as his home life was falling apart. Dr. Sheila Ashtiju addressed this by prescribing testosterone, but ALSO by giving him supplements to build up his adrenal glands naturally. The goal would eventually be that Rick would require less of this testosterone cream and that his body would resume making it on its own. (This two-pronged approach to sexual dysfunction is truly what separates mediocre MD's from excellent ones. I know a few people who practice medicine the way that Dr. Sheila does. They are not always easy to find, but they are out there!)

Rick's sexual vigor returns when he embraces exercise, weight loss, the use of testosterone and has more restorative sleep. He finds an outlet for his improved erections in the motel with various women. The importance of this part of the story is that we get to learn a few things. First, Rick has returned to his ability to have ALL forms of sex, including penetrative sex, and not just masturbation. Secondly, it has taken Rick over a year to achieve full recovery from his erectile dysfunction. This type of treatment is not a quick fix, but his weight loss and glances from women at the grocery store are enough motivation to keep Rick on this path, even though he knows he will not likely reestablish any sex with his wife. Finally, Rick's ability to have sex again gives him the necessary courage to leave a loveless marriage. While this is not the happiest of endings, it does unveil the power of a bodily system that is responding naturally to sexual urges and the spill-over effect that overall health can bring to the mind.

In short, Rick's erectile dysfunction is not simply cured by Cialis. The return of Rick's sex drive is hard-won. It is not a simple undertaking and it forces him to look at several areas of his life that need to change. There are many ways to treat erectile dysfunction. But the most effective ones are those that encompass a holistic approach, much like the one that Dr. Sheila Ashtiju endorses. Even though Dr. Ashtiju believes that she envies the sexual response in men, that it is so easy, so "cut and dry", it is from Rick that we learn how complicated and miraculous a simple erection can be.

Suggestions for men like Rick with erectile dysfunction include the following:

1.  Get daily exercise and keep your weight down.
2.  Try to manage life stress.
3.  Get more sleep.

4.  If you are interested in having your testosterone level checked, find a medical specialist who is skilled in bioidentical hormone replacement.
5.  Examine what you want out of your sex life and then communicate with your partner in how to get it.

# Kirk

Kirk's story is unfortunately quite typical of young men with pelvic pain. This type of patient often has little to no access to medical care, nor does he have knowledge of his condition. Kirk's story starts as he is drumming in the band and working as a bartender. He develops symptoms of urinary urgency and pain but has not the first idea why. Nor does the only doctor that he visits at the clinic that specializes in Sexually Transmitted Infections. At first, Kirk hopes that his penile pain is a result of chlamydia. This is because chlamydia is treated with the use of antibiotics and is highly curable.

Kirk finds that he has no actual diagnosis for his pelvic pain. There is no distinct provoking factor or event, no bacteria or infection to pin his symptoms upon. This is uniquely distressing to any person. Kirk's symptoms then begin to interfere with his sexual life. He has pain in his testicles after sex and at one point in the book describes newly developed premature ejaculation. What Kirk does not realize is that he displays many of the classic symptoms of Chronic Pelvic Pain Syndrome. This is a term used to describe pain that can affect the penis, testicles and rectum. The muscles of the pelvic floor in men are the ones that would be in contact with the saddle of a horse. These very muscles are the ones responsible for urination, ejaculation and defecation. Research suggests that pain in this region can tighten the pelvic floor musculature and often result in discomfort associated with these bodily functions. (Faubion, 2012)

Normal urination requires that the bladder and pelvic floor muscles, or "saddle region", must relax in order to allow urine to flow out of the urethra. Kirk cannot produce a urine sample for the doctor at the clinic for Sexually Transmitted Infections because he is clenching his saddle muscles so tightly that urine cannot flow out naturally. The tension in these saddle muscles creates pain along the urethra and often mimics symptoms of a urinary tract infection or STI, though Rick has neither. Towards the end of Kirk's story, he finds that he leaks urine when he works out in the cold at the gas station. Many men with tight pelvic floor muscles have urinary hesitancy, dribbling and leakage, all from a poorly coordinated pattern of their muscles not being able to lengthen enough to allow all the urine to be drained from the bladder "in one sitting". Speaking of sitting, Kirk also notes that he is able to void urine with more ease when he is sitting down on the toilet versus standing up. This is usually the first technique that pelvic floor physical therapists teach men to employ when they have urinary symptoms. It works because the butt cheeks, or gluteal muscles are not gripping together and preventing urine from exiting the bladder, as they are when a man stands at a urinal. The bladder can fully relax in the seated position, all the urine will escape the bladder "in one sitting" and this will prevent both urinary hesitancy and difficulty starting a urinary stream, as well as urinary dribbling and leakage.

Why does Kirk have pain with sex? Why does he want to grab his scrotum after ejaculation and scream, when sex is a pleasurable activity for most men? This is a symptom of men with tight pelvic floor muscles. The typical response of the body during arousal is pooling of blood in the perineum, around the testicles and up into the penis. For men with tight muscles in this area of the body, their taut muscular tissue prevents the engorgement of the penis and testicles. Blood enters this "saddle region" of the groin, but because the tissues are unable to stretch and accommodate that rush of blood which is necessary to enhance an erection, pain, spasm and erectile dysfunction are the result. In sum, men with these symptoms of Chronic Pelvic Pain Syndrome often have pain associated with arousal and ejaculation. Some men have pain which lasts hours after climax, to the point where they avoid sex altogether.

Many men with these symptoms will try just about anything to stop the pain in their saddle regions. Especially if they have not been diagnosed with something concrete and then offered treatment. At first, Kirk tries to stop his pain by drinking. This is initially effective, but in time, he notices that when he gets very drunk, the pain in his pelvis worsens with his hangover. From a medical standpoint, why would drinking excessive amounts of alcohol worsen pelvic pain? There are two main reasons. The first is that alcohol dehydrates the body and causes the urinary stream to flow less freely and urine then becomes very concentrated and dark in color. The second reason that alcohol would worsen pelvic pain in Kirk's case is because alcohol is highly irritating to the walls of the bladder. It creates an acidic environment therein which manifests with pain in the lower abdomen and along the urethra.

Marijuana is what Kirk also uses to quell his pain. This is somewhat helpful to him, as it can be to others with Chronic Pelvic Pain Syndrome, because it creates some degree of full body and mind relaxation, which alcohol does not. Medical marijuana is now being prescribed for patients with Chronic Pelvic Pain Syndrome and the results are positive. Notice that when things are going well for Kirk, when his band gets the offer to go on tour, he ceases drinking temporarily. He even goes running through the streets of Manhattan and forgets that he ever had pelvic pain at all. The sudden disappearance of pelvic pain is also common in these men. The pain waxes and wanes, like the tide. Stressful life events will often usher the pelvic pain back. And just as the band gets on the road and the drug and heavy alcohol use resumes, Kirk's symptoms return with a vengeance. He finds that he can no longer sit on his drummer's stool for too long, because it worsens the pain. Seated pain is also a common finding in men with Chronic Pelvic Pain Syndrome. Pain with prolonged sitting causes the small saddle muscles to shorten and tighten.

There is a point in Kirk's story when he notices that he no longer has erections in the morning. This is consistent with his medical problem. And here's why: the average male has between three to five spontaneous erections through the course of one evening of sleep. These nocturnal erections last approximately 30 minutes and occur because the spinal nerves send calming signals into the pelvis, causing the penis and testicles to become engorged with blood. Most men are not aware that they are having these erections. They are a sign of a healthy pelvic floor and a relaxed nervous system. In the case of Kirk and many guys with pain in the saddle region, the mechanism of the spine which sends the signal to increase blood flow to the groin is disrupted. Kirk's nervous system is on overload because of his pain and the anxiety that surrounds his pain, and it never slows down in sleep to allow these evening erections. Furthermore, because of his boozing, drug use and partying lifestyle, Kirk is not likely getting any deep sleep, which also prevents his nervous system from quieting.

For men who want to know if they are having nocturnal erections, there are two methods to find out. The first is the Stamp Method. It is rather primitive (said in the words of my patients) and requires a roll of stamps that have dried glue on the back that one would have to moisten with saliva to adhere to an envelope. The stamps that are actual stickers will not work for this. The test involves wrapping a few stamps around the base of the penis before sleep, securing them in a circle, and then checking the circle of stamps that surround the penis in the morning. In theory, the increasing girth of the penis during a nocturnal erection would break the circle of stamps and offer proof that at least one erection had occurred during the sleep cycle. If the circle of stamps remains intact at the base of the penis, the man *may not* have had an erection. There are many things wrong with this test, most notably the fact that it is very difficult to purchase this type of stamp these days. Another practical failure of this test in being accurate is if the man simply rolled over in his sleep, causing the circle of stamps to break, without any actual erection having taken place.

A more scientific method of studying nocturnal erections has emerged. Known as the RigiScan™, there is a portable home device used to evaluate the quality of nighttime erections. This is a small battery-operated unit which gets strapped to a man's thigh. It is equipped with two loops, one of which goes around the base of the penis, and the other wraps around the area just underneath the glans penis. Throughout the night, this device measures the amount of blood flow into the penis and the rigidity of a man's erections. This test is repeated several nights in a row and the data is stored on the device so that a man's physician can access it. A test like this would help a man with Chronic Pelvic Pain Syndrome to know where he is in the process of recovery from his diagnosis. This is because once severe pelvic pain is managed with this condition, the evening and morning erections would likely return. Wouldn't it have been of great assistance for Kirk to have access to information and technology like this to help him understand what was happening in his body?

Sadly, many men out in the world are suffering from the various symptoms of Chronic Pelvic Pain Syndrome without the access to medical care or information to help them. The character of Kirk was written to give a voice to these nameless guys. While he does get some assistance in his recovery from drug addiction, Kirk is left hanging when it comes to his pelvic problems. The ending of Kirk's story was intended to shed light on what happens when unmitigated pain storms through the body and how it impacts the brain and relationships.

It is difficult to know how many men are living with Chronic Pelvic Pain Syndrome. This is because many men with these symptoms wait for years before going to see a physician. And often when they do, their doctors have not heard of this diagnosis and fail to direct their patients in the right direction to manage the symptoms. It is my sincere hope that more awareness can be spread about this problem. As a physical therapist, I treat more men than I can count who feel isolated, anxious and depressed as they live in secret pain which society does not acknowledge.

Below is a list of medical conditions that may predispose men to developing the symptoms of Chronic Pelvic Pain Syndrome:

1. Lyme disease
2. A history of kidney stones
3. A previous history of surgeries including appendix removal, hernia repair or a total hip replacement
4. Hip osteoarthritis or a tear of the labrum of the hip
5. Low back pain
6. Fibromyalgia or Chronic Fatigue Syndrome
7. A previously contracted Sexually Transmitted Infection
8. Migraine Headaches or Temporomandibular Joint Pain (jaw pain)

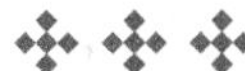

# Sheila

Dr. Sheila Ashtiju begins her medical career working for a major medical institution in Texas. She rises in her skill of treating prostate cancer, she wins awards and is well-celebrated and respected as a urologist. Sheila then tires of performing prostate removals and she looks for a change in vocation that will lead to more personal meaning for her.

Sheila decides to move to another state and opens her own practice to treat male sexual health. She does not accept payment from health insurance companies and relies on her patients paying out of pocket to get their problems addressed. She is pleasantly surprised to discover that she has a waiting list of several months of men who seek out her specialty. Part of what makes practitioners like Dr. Sheila Ashtiju so unique is that they are able to draw from whatever sources of treatment that they see fit. In other words, if Sheila was working for the hospital in Houston, she would be under the parameters of the hospital network to tell her how long she could spend with each patient and what pharmaceutical agents she could prescribe to her patients. Hospital networks often prescribe medications that have been approved by the Food and Drug Administration. Any drug approved by the FDA must undergo rigorous testing and clinical trials to ensure that the drug is deemed "safe". Yet how many times have we all seen commercials on the television featuring a group of lawyers willing to represent anyone who has taken a certain drug, because of some dreadful side-effects that were only discovered years later?

Sheila is willing to go outside of the norms of American medicine to tap into the healing powers of her patients. Remember when she prescribed Rick the natural adrenal supplement to boost his body's ability to make its own cortisol? She also prescribed him testosterone cream to apply to his testicles each night. These kinds of hormones are called "bioidentical". This means that the hormones of testosterone, progesterone and estrogen can be formulated to mimic exactly the hormones as they are naturally produced by the human body. This type of hormone replacement therapy is coming into vogue, as the general public is leery of the use of synthesized hormones that are manufactured by pharmaceutical companies.

Bioidentical hormones are typically made in a compounding pharmacy. These hormones are mixed into creams which maximize absorption by the body. Health insurance companies do not usually cover the cost of these creams. This is likely because there are not a lot of studies on the benefits/risks of bioidentical hormones. There are not a lot of studies – because Big Pharma does not stand to make as much profit off bioidentical hormones, as they do from synthesized hormones like the birth control pill for women.

One can see why finding a physician like Dr. Sheila Ashtiju would offer something apart from going to a urologist who works out of a hospital conglomerate. Sheila is able to treat the root cause of Rick's erectile dysfunction. She doesn't give him Cialis, because he doesn't need it. He just needs his body to return to a level of equilibrium wherein sex would be a natural inclination.

Notice how Sheila is also able to treat her own lack of sexual appetite. She prescribes herself progesterone cream to be applied to her forearms around the time of ovulation in her menstrual cycle. Progesterone is the "let's get laid" hormone for women (my gynecologist's turn of phrase) and it is produced around ovulation to make a woman crave sex, thus furthering her chances of getting pregnant when her egg is ready to be fertilized. Testosterone is also produced in women in very small doses, and it does increase libido, as it does in men. Sheila prescribes herself some of that cream to be applied to her vulva to heighten her sexual response.

In time, Sheila's sexual desire returns. She accomplishes this by boosting her body's resources to bring herself back into hormonal balance. Sheila is also aware as to *why* her sex drive plummeted. This is because she had been under extreme stress from having moved away from her family, opening her own business and having very little exposure to the natural sunlight under which she had spent most of her life. Anxiety and stress will decrease the sex drives of both men and women. Why? Because from an evolutionary perspective, sex is a *pleasant little extra* that the body can enjoy once the survival needs of food, shelter and protection are already met. It isn't ideal for a couple to get pregnant during a famine, and their bodies know this.

There are physicians out there who treat their patients and themselves in precisely the way that Dr. Sheila Ashtiju does. They often do not accept health insurance plans and they will likely prescribe hormones or supplements that are not covered by insurance. This raises the question as to whether Rick would have gotten better had he gone to a traditional urologist. He certainly might have. It would have cost him less money and he would have been prescribed Cialis, Viagra or Levitra and been able to have sex. But would that quick fix have led Rick down the road of embracing his overall health? In treating many Ricks through the years as a physical therapist, I do not think that Rick would have recovered nearly as well without Sheila. The patients who make lifestyle changes and commit to a trajectory of good health almost always fare better than the ones who believe that one pill or intervention will be their personal game-changer.

Tips for men with erectile dysfunction:

1. While hormone deficits are not always the primary cause of sexual dysfunction, it may interest you to have your hormone levels checked. If so, find a doctor who is experienced with and feels comfortable prescribing bioidentical hormones.
2. Manage high blood pressure and diabetes as well as you can, as both contribute to erectile dysfunction.
3. Remember that erectile dysfunction will usually get worse during difficult and stressful times; give your body a break when this happens and don't feel badly about it. When the stressful trigger in your life is resolved, you may notice a spontaneous return in your sex drive.

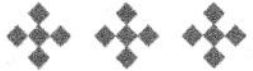

# Tom

Tom represents a man who has been diagnosed with Chronic Pelvic Pain Syndrome. The symptoms of Chronic Pelvic Pain include the following: 1) urinary hesitancy, pain or urgency 2) pain with sex 3) rectal pain, spasms and constipation and 4) pain with sitting. Tom has pain with sex, he has rectal spasms and constipation, and sitting for long periods of time on an airplane make his symptoms worse. Notice that he is spared the urinary symptoms that Kirk experiences while on tour with his band. Such variability among men with this diagnosis is common. In other words, some men can have pain-free sex but have rectal pain. Others have urinary dribbling and discomfort when sitting but they have no bowel or sexual problems. Some men have all four of the classic signs of CPPS as listed above. Chronic Pelvic Pain Syndrome is a usually a cluster of these problems with multi-dimensional effects for each patient.

Tom's journey begins with severe pelvic pain which he attempts to deal with himself. He uses wine as anesthetic, but he realizes that it is ineffective. Tom calls a urologist and makes an appointment. Tom is told upon his first exam with the urologist that he has "prostatitis". This is a diagnosis that is often used by urologists to explain rectal pain and pain which extends into the pelvic floor, testicles and penis. The theory behind the diagnosis is that the prostate gland becomes inflamed and thereby causes the pelvic pain. Tom is doubtful of both the care that he gets from the young urologist and the diagnosis of "prostatitis". The doctor gives Tom an antibiotic to treat bacteria in his prostate and a steroid to calm the inflammation in his saddle region.

In the world of pelvic floor physical therapy, we often treat men who have been given this diagnosis of "prostatitis". They usually are prescribed some oral antibiotics, often more than one round of a given type. Tom does not like this treatment idea, and he is wise to question it. In an article written in the *World Journal of Urology,* only about 5% of men who are given the diagnosis of prostatitis have positive cultures of bacteria in the prostate. (Potts, 2003) An article published only five years later in 2008 found that despite the evidence that antibiotics are not effective in treating these symptoms of chronic pelvic pain, they are prescribed to 69% of men. (Taylor, 2008) So, what does this tell us? Why are these men who are suffering from pelvic pain given a diagnosis which suggests that they have an infection, bacteria or inflammation of their prostates, when there is so little research to support it?

Tom decides not to take the advice of his urologist and looks for another professional. Tom finds Dr. Nathan Shah. Dr. Shah very quickly asks Tom a series of questions and surmises that his patient does *not* require the administration of antibiotics for an infection that may or may not exist. Instead, Tom needs his pain to be controlled by a series of injections to the tight muscles of his pelvic floor, which thereby decrease the tension of these muscles and decrease the symptoms of constipation and painful sex. Tom's discovery of a practitioner who listens to him and treats him according to his actual symptoms have a profound impact on his life. It is after meeting Dr. Nathan Shah that Tom drives home to his wife and admits to her why he has been avoiding sex.

Not only does Dr. Shah offer injections to help Tom, but he also suggests some lifestyle modifications. Yoga and meditation have excellent results for patients like Tom. Towards the end of Tom's story, he goes to the meditation chapel of the airport before each flight to calm his mind. He uses a specialized seat cushion which has a cut-out in the middle to avoid any direct pressure to his sore saddle muscles. Tom also takes Dr. Shah's suggestion to find a pelvic floor physical therapist. It is through these treatments with his pelvic floor PT that Tom is awakened to the connection between his tight muscles and pelvic pain.

For patients with pelvic pain and the symptoms of Chronic Pelvic Pain Syndrome, they are often helped by stretching and release to these muscles. I have seen it personally in the clinic where I work, but don't just take my word for it. In a study performed in 2005, men who were diagnosed with Chronic Pelvic Pain Syndrome participated in a protocol that included hands-on trigger point release to the abdomen and perineum performed by physical therapists. A global improvement in pain and urinary symptoms occurred for 72% of the participants of the study. (Anderson, 2005)

Pelvic floor physical therapy is extremely beneficial for men with pelvic pain. However, it often takes men a while to show up at the physical therapist's office. This may largely be due to the fact that many urologists are not yet aware of how helpful a modality this can be to their patients. It may also be driven by fear and a sense of shame men have when something is wrong with their penises. Men often come to pelvic floor PT when they have exhausted all other medical options, or they don't feel as though anyone is listening to them. Once the initial indignity of the physical therapy evaluation is conquered, men are often quite open about their symptoms and feel relieved to have a sounding board for their pain. Yes, this does require that a therapist places a finger inside the rectum to assess the tension of the pelvic floor muscles. The rationale for this is *not* to weigh in on the status, size or feel of the prostate gland; rather, it is the simplest way for the physical therapist to release the muscles that are holding on for dear life and causing the urinary, sexual and bowel related symptoms. After the first few times of enduring this treatment, many men report not minding it at all, because the relief they experience thereafter is nothing short of remarkable.

There is a lot more that goes into treating men with this condition than a finger in the bum. Pelvic floor PT's spend a lot of time employing relaxation techniques, such as skin rolling of the abdomen, yoga, stretching and deep breathing with their patients. A lot of education is involved, and just as Tom's physical therapist was able to help him to address his chronic constipation, we pelvic floor therapists shy away at nothing in order to help our patients get well. Once something like constipation or urinary pain is under control, sex can become a pleasurable and pain-free activity once more. Remember, we are treating the muscles that control all three of the bodily functions of urination, sex and defecation. These functions must take place within a very small bony cavity within the pelvis. When one of the functions is impaired, the other ones may feel askew as well. Our goal is to help our patients rebalance their pelvises and to allow health and natural function to be restored.

A pivotal part of pelvic floor physical therapy is biofeedback. While this was not mentioned in Tom's tale of his time in physical therapy (as Tom's story was complicated and I did not want to add so many details as to confuse the reader), biofeedback involves placing sensors on either side of the rectum. These sensors are connected to a computer screen. The patient is asked to both contract and relax his pelvic floor muscles. He can see on the computer screen what level of activity his muscles are putting forth. For a man with tight pelvic floor muscles, this is a powerful tool to allow him to ascertain where his pelvic floor muscles are and what he can do to relax them. Many patients have no idea how much tension they are holding in their saddles until they see it on the computer screen and can perform positioning, breathing techniques and stretches to bring that tension down. The treatment technique of biofeedback is well-documented in medical literature in assisting men to decrease pelvic floor tightness. (Tries, 2005)

On a final note, some physicians are prescribing suppositories for men with pelvic pain. Not all MD's are on board with this treatment, as there are not enough studies to support them. Valium is a benzodiazepine which works as a tranquilizer, but also as an effective muscle relaxant. It is because of these muscle relaxing properties that Valium is sometimes used as a suppository and placed within the rectum at night. The theory behind this treatment is that the medication would relax the muscles locally at the level of the pelvic floor, thereby allowing the patient to awaken in the morning with far less tension. These suppositories are compounded in smaller pharmacies. Many insurance companies do not cover them. Furthermore, the risk versus benefit ratio may not be sufficient to warrant an MD prescribing a controlled substance in this fashion.

Cannabis is beginning to be used to treat pelvic pain as well. This is the non-hallucinogenic portion of the marijuana plant. Some patients have found relief when taking CBD oil orally, rubbing it on their perineums for local pain control or using rectal suppositories. My patients have reported some relief from these products; however, a dearth of research is hindering more expansive use of CBD oil in the medical world at this time.

Thoughts for men who have been diagnosed with Chronic Pelvic Pain Syndrome:

1. Find a urologist who acknowledges your condition. Don't stay with one urologist if you don't feel listened to.
2. Engage in any activity of mindfulness to help calm the brain: meditation, yoga, being in nature.
3. Go to a pelvic floor physical therapist. You will learn about your diagnosis and play an active role in your own recovery.
4. Be patient with yourself. Your symptoms may not go away overnight, but increased awareness of your body will bring improved results.

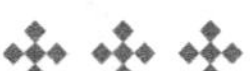

# Oliver

Oliver is upset when his primary doctor suggests that he might have some substantial risk factors for prostate cancer. While the doctor's delivery of this information is insensitive, labeling Oliver as an "African-American" when he is, in fact, Jamaican, the doctor is correct in picking up on some significant risk factors that Oliver has in developing this type of cancer. Black men have the highest risk of developing prostate cancer, followed next by white men and then Hispanics. The risk is lowest for men from the Pacific Islands, Asia and Native Americans. While Oliver is young to be diagnosed with prostate cancer, he has another major risk factor, because his father also has prostate cancer. Having one first-degree relative with this disease doubles the risk of developing it. Oliver is only in his forties and the average age of this diagnosis is usually between 65-70. Yet with this genetic combination, Oliver is one of the men who gets the disease earlier in his life. (Ferlay, 2010)

Oliver's doctor discovers that his patient has an elevated PSA level. The acronym PSA stands for a Prostate Specific Antigen, which is a protein produced by the cells of the prostate that form the liquid secreted by the prostate during ejaculation. It is standard practice for physicians to look at this PSA level in the blood. There are normal values, but if an MD notices that this number is elevated, or that it rapidly increases from year to year, this may be an indicator of prostate cancer. The PSA is not really a gold-standard of diagnosis, because a man's PSA levels can be higher than normal for a number of reasons that often have nothing to do with the presence of cancer cells. This is why a biopsy is usually performed on the prostate if a PSA level is deemed high. If there are no cancer cells within the prostate upon biopsy, then most doctors will simply track the PSA levels from year to year. If cancer cells are discovered in the prostate, as they were in Oliver, there are treatments available.

Oliver's father had radioactive seeds implanted in his pelvis, around the location of his prostate. This low-dose radiation is called brachytherapy and is used for men with prostate cancer at certain stages of the disease. It is an effective form of treatment, with the most notable side-effects being urinary incontinence or erectile dysfunction. Sometimes these side-effects are temporary and resolve. Other times, men need to rely on urinary pads and the use of medication to address their erectile dysfunction. Another type of radiation therapy is given to a man's prostate via an external beam laser. Again, the idea is to irradiate the tissues around the prostate to demolish the cancer cells therein. One of the unfortunate side-effects of this treatment technique, or any use of radiation, is that healthy tissue is also destroyed. That said, radiation is often the go-to treatment for many men over sixty with prostate cancer, and the success rates in destroying the cancerous cells are quite high these days.

Oliver's urologist does not want to use radiation on his patient. Rather, he suggests removal of the prostate, or prostatectomy. One of the reasons that this urologist prefers removal of the organ which has cancer is because of Oliver's young age and how aggressive his cancer presents. With more aggressive prostate cancer and a younger age of diagnosis, many doctors prefer this surgery to radiation, in the effort to get all the cancer cells removed from the body and to prevent the cancer cells from spreading to the surrounding lymph nodes or bladder. Furthermore, once radiation is delivered to the prostate, a surgical removal of the gland will be much more complicated, as the tissues which are bombarded by the radiation are now fragile and less elastic. The side-effects of a prostatectomy, or prostate removal, are usually urinary incontinence and erectile dysfunction. Oliver reports both in the beginning of his recovery after surgery, but both are resolved within a matter of a few months. Typical resolution of these side-effects takes up to two years, and full recovery is possible. Men are infertile after a prostatectomy and have dry ejaculate, as there is no liquid produced by the prostate to carry the sperm through the head of the penis. Many patients report the same sensation of climax, however, and are able to get an erection rigid enough to allow for penetrative sex.

The surgical removal of the prostate gland is typically done in one of two ways. It can be performed in the traditional open-surgical fashion, with an incision made either to the perineum or on the lower belly. Another more recent surgical option is via laparoscopy. This is an operation that uses small incisions in the skin and a guided camera to remove the tissues in question. In the case of prostate cancer, these incisions are made along the abdomen and are used as portals of entry for the surgeon to go in and carefully dissect the tissues without making larger cuts through muscles. A laparoscopic radical prostatectomy is now often performed with the assistance of a robot with voice-controlled arms that the surgeon can utilize.

In treating men immediately after a prostatectomy, many of them avoid sexual activity. This may be due to the fear of urinary leakage during the act of sex, which can resolve in time. Men are usually given medical clearance to resume sexual activity merely four weeks after surgery. They are often prescribed Cialis, Levitra or Viagra. This is helpful not only to allow men to engage in sex, but these pharmaceuticals flood the penis and testicles with blood, thereby facilitating natural healing to occur. Pelvic floor physical therapists encourage their patients to return to sex and have it often. Initially, many men are uncomfortable surrounding sex during this process after surgery, but the ones who return to sex more readily have better long-term outcomes of sexual satisfaction following removal of the prostate.

Pelvic floor physical therapy can be extremely beneficial for men after removal of the prostate. While Oliver did not undergo pelvic floor PT, there is significant research to back up the importance of receiving this type of treatment to decrease the side-effects of the surgery. In a study performed by Van Kampen, men who performed pelvic floor exercises after a prostate removal achieved urinary continence sooner than the control group who did not. (Van Kampen, 2000) A much more recent study observed an improvement of 75.6% in urinary leakage in men who engaged in a pelvic floor physical therapy program for three months following a prostatectomy. (Sathianathen, 2017) Another study weighed in on erectile dysfunction and the efficacy of pelvic floor physical therapy following prostate removal. This research showed that 40% of men with erectile dysfunction after prostate removal returned to normal erectile function, and another 35.5% of the patients reported continued improvement of the sexual response after completion of six months of pelvic floor exercises. (Dorey, 2004)

What does this tell us? That strengthening and coordinating the pelvic floor muscles has a clear link to decreasing urinary leakage and improving erections. A further benefit to receiving pelvic floor PT after a diagnosis of prostate cancer is to have a sounding board to frankly discuss concerns surrounding these issues. Who else can a guy talk to about such things? Your urologist won't likely have the time. Many psychologists are not aware of these unwanted side-effects of prostate cancer. And your partner may not fully grasp what you are going through.

The vast majority of men return to work within 12 months of having received treatment for prostate cancer. Work fulfills many purposes including financial reward, social interaction, a sense of routine, and some men describe work as their "life" or "family". While they are not thrilled about the social stigma associated with this type of cancer and may not discuss their diagnosis with coworkers, going back to work offers these guys a sense of normalcy. (Grunfeld, 2013) This is a powerful statistic which underlines the importance that men place on being providers and their desire to be part of the commerce of the world in which they live.

Another form of prostate cancer treatment is a pharmaceutical intervention known as Androgen Deprivation Therapy. These are medications which are used to suppress testosterone production, as there have been older studies linking testosterone to the growth of cancer cells in the prostate. The rationale behind this treatment is that a lack of testosterone in the body will shrink the cancer and prevent it from spreading. This serves as an explanation as to why men with a prostate cancer diagnosis are not prescribed testosterone for their erectile dysfunction; it isn't used as it was for Rick the plumber to increase sexual drive.

Androgen Deprivation Therapy certainly has its place. It has been scientifically proven to shrink cancer cells within the prostate and is an alternative to surgery or radiation for men with prostate cancer. Some doctors also use Androgen Deprivation Therapy in conjunction with radiation to keep the cancer from returning. It should be noted, however, that reducing testosterone in males from a medical standpoint comes with significant costs to men's overall health. Some side-effects include lowered libido, hot flashes, loss of bone density, loss of muscle mass and a decrease in physical strength.

I'd like to go out on a limb here and cite some new research that has made its way into the world of prostate health. Conventional wisdom and previous scientific studies suggested that testosterone feeds prostate cancer cells. In an article published as recently as 2015, scientific literature was analyzed to determine if testosterone replacement used under a physician's guidance either increased a man's chance of acquiring prostate cancer later in life or if testosterone used after a prostate cancer diagnosis would worsen or grow the disease. Two things were discovered: 1) Men who underwent hormone replacement were NOT more likely to get a diagnosis of prostate cancer down the road and 2) Men who received testosterone therapy for non-aggressive and well-localized prostate cancer did NOT show higher rates of recurrence of cancer or worse outcomes than those who did not receive testosterone replacement. (Kaplan, 2015) While this research is quite new and further studies are warranted, if I was a guy who was diagnosed with prostate cancer that was well-controlled,

I would want to find a urologist who was curious about this controversial change in how to manage prostate cancer; if only because of the positive effects of maintaining safe testosterone levels for general health and well-being.

Finally, there are a growing number of urologists who see slow-growing prostate cancers in men over sixty which do not present with many symptoms. These urologists are offering two noninvasive treatments to track the cancer. The first is called Active Surveillance. In this case, the cancer within the prostate will be left alone, but the patient will return to his physician every 6 months for a Prostate Specific Antigen test and a biopsy can be performed every 1 to 3 years. These measures are taken to ensure that the prostate cancer is not growing. The second treatment type is known as Watchful Waiting, where there is even less testing involved, and the patient simply monitors any change in his symptoms. Because prostate cancer has a low mortality rate (especially if it is a non-aggressive form), some men opt to avoid surgery and radiation, due to the side-effects of erectile dysfunction and urinary leakage. This is favored by older men who feel comfortable with managing the disease rather than trying to cure it.

This book is written from the point of view of a pelvic floor physical therapist in helping men recover after a diagnosis prostate cancer. I haven't delved into the vast amount of information that exists on this subject, because in the words of many of my college professors, that would be "beyond the scope of this course". This nonfiction explanation about Oliver is a way to bring the science into view to better understand why he was diagnosed as he was, why he avoided sex immediately after surgery and how he was able to live a good life without a prostate.

Tips for men who have been diagnosed with prostate cancer:

1. Get treatment opinions from more than one urologist. This condition is treated in many ways, and only you know which treatment will be right for you.

2. Find a pelvic floor physical therapist. It will be helpful to go for *at least* one session before surgery or treatment (more than one session would be better) to get a sense of where your pelvic floor muscles are and what they do. You can learn how to do Kegel exercises (they aren't just for women). Pelvic floor PT will also be extremely beneficial after your treatment to prevent urinary leakage and improve sexual function.

3. Buy a book entitled *Prostate Recovery Map: Men's Action Plan 2* (Allingham, 2017) The author is named Craig Allingham and he is a pelvic floor physiotherapist in Australia. This is a how-to guide for strengthening the pelvic floor and what to expect with a diagnosis of prostate cancer. This book is wonderfully simple and yet it covers a lot of ground. It is also light-hearted in discussing a heavy topic.

4. Know that prostate cancer is the second most commonly diagnosed type of cancer in the United States, with skin cancer being the first. There are many other men out there just like you. This is a treatable cancer and your odds for longevity and pelvic health after treatment are extremely high.

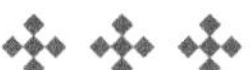

# Part III

# The Back Story

*"I'm not one for easy."* Henry Rolnik, a Polish rebel who escaped a Nazi prison camp

When I graduated from physical therapy school with my master's degree in 1998, there were no physical therapy jobs to be found. I had attended college in Philadelphia and during that time, my parents had relocated to Pittsburgh, Pennsylvania. I had no affiliation with the city of Pittsburgh, but without a job, I did what any 23-year-old without a career does; I moved in with my parents. It was in late September when I drove from Philadelphia to Pittsburgh in a small Honda Civic hatchback that my father had purchased for me. I recall that drive along the Pennsylvania Turnpike. It was long and dull, unmarked by anything other than my own dull shame in having failed to secure employment after graduating from college.

Fall very quickly morphed into winter. The sun did not emerge from the grey sky of Pittsburgh. Weeks turned into months, and snow fell hard upon the land of Western Pennsylvania. By the time Christmas came, there was a 2-inch-thick coating of ice that covered the sidewalks of Pittsburgh. It did not melt until late spring. My Mom and I argued about stupid things, like when I left the garage door open or used too much parmesan cheese when cooking pasta with olive oil. My Dad looked at us, grown women who should have navigated a better way to live together, and I still wonder what he thought about why we didn't. It was such a hard winter.

I recall buying gasoline from a small corner store in Pittsburgh that was Russian-owned. Unlike in New Jersey, which is one of the two states in America that have attendants to pump gasoline for their customers (we are so spoiled here), I had to pump my own gasoline. It was always a frigid day, in a not-so-safe area that I used to get the gasoline to fuel my little Honda. My father went there often, and he liked the proprietors of the establishment who wore fur black hats. My Dad called it "The Russian Tea Room". There was a bullet-proof clear shield that protected the Russians from bad customers. We had to put our cash or credit card into a metal drawer and then push the drawer into a secure little stand where the Russians collected our money for the gasoline we would buy.

There was one day that was so very cold that I remarked to the man in the black fur hat, "It is freezing today. How can you stand this weather?" The Russian man smiled and laughed. I could hear him through the bullet-proof glass. "My dear, I am from Siberia! To me, this weather is *children's game!*" I tucked that memory away, as I got back in my little Honda. It was not until 15 years later that the Russian man's words rang so very true.

I have since made peace with the city of Pittsburgh. I located the characters of Rick and Sheila in precisely that geographical area. It was never the city's fault that I was placed under her grey skies. I was unable to see the beauty of the Steel City at that time. Because of my life circumstances, age, and immaturity, I had written off Pittsburgh like a bad relationship. And I was wrong to do so. It has taken some time to remember the words of the man from the "Russian Tea Room"; to acknowledge that we all need darkness and some ice on the ground to draw inwards, to see the very hard things that we wish were not right in front of us.

In working with men who have pelvic pain, I am often reminded of the words of the Russian man from the gasoline station. When I asked him if the cold bothered him, the man replied, "I am from Siberia. To me, this weather is *children's game!*" For people suffering from low back pain, a rotator cuff tear, or a herniation of a disc in the neck, this pain is very real. As a physical therapist, I have seen what chronic pain can do to an individual. However, pelvic pain is vastly different from other types of musculoskeletal pain. This is because pelvic pain affects the bodily functions of urination, sex and bowel movements. All three of these bodily functions are important to daily living. Not being able to pee, have sex, or crap in a normal way is terrifying and awful.

Living with chronic pain of any kind is challenging. Yet living with chronic *pelvic* pain makes other kinds of musculoskeletal problems seem like child's play; or as the Russian gas attendant said so well, *children's game.* As for the stories that are in this book, they are completely fictional. These characters do, however, represent and are a compilation of the many stories I have heard from the multitudes of men I have treated. Their symptoms are crippling, but their recovery from these symptoms is redeeming.

The characters of Rick, Kirk, Sheila, Tom and Oliver are all invented. But the difficulties they each endure are very real. In writing about pelvic pain and cancer, I wanted to create people with whom the reader could resonate. I wanted the world to understand how the diagnosis of pelvic dysfunction has such far-reaching implications. These characters were made-up to help get inside the minds of these four men and their female physician. If a guy with pelvic pain dreads having sex with his partner, he will avoid his partner and snap at his children, without meaning to do so. If a man suddenly gets diagnosed with prostate cancer when he has no symptoms and is an upstanding sharpshooter for the U.S. Army, he will want to go out and hunt to kill anything in his path.

When I was finished writing the first part of the book with the fictional stories, I missed all five characters deeply. In my head, they had become real. I worried about them, I wondered what they were thinking or doing. This last portion of the book is meant to illuminate where these five people came from and why they are so important to the topic of this book. This is the backstory. Perhaps it all started during my own drive to Pittsburgh. At that time, I could not appreciate the beauty of the winding passage through the Allegheny Mountains, nor the charms of Pittsburgh at the end of the journey. The Pennsylvania Turnpike had been miles of pavement then. I began my journey in much the same way as these characters did: in the thick of great boredom, ennui and turmoil, blind to what is in front of them, until they each emerge from their own Fort Pitt Tunnel to find mental and physical healing, out of the enclosed darkness and into the sunlight.

# Rick

Rick is a quintessential blue-collar guy. He takes enormous pride in his work and has a great deal of respect for his own father, who gave him the plumbing business. Rick is also a fair and compassionate man. He does work for his customers who don't have much money and doesn't charge them full price. Rick is a loyal husband throughout most of his marriage. It isn't until he becomes the caretaker for his ill wife that he starts noticing his problem of erectile dysfunction.

Rick's story begins as his wife Nicole tells him that sex is off the table in their marriage. He gets into his hot tub and cannot achieve any semblance of an erection. From this point forward, Nicole becomes more and more withdrawn. Rick becomes her primary caretaker, while he also pursues a path to rediscover his own sexual desire.

Once Rick finds a solution to his erectile problems, he does what seems unthinkable. Rick finds women online and meets them for sex in a local motel *(with hourly rates, at that)*. Rick has a fair amount of shame in what he is doing. While he is a bit disappointed in himself, he is also exhibiting the behavior of any sexually virile human when denied sex for protracted periods of time. Rick has been given a taste of what great sex is like, after years of anxiety and the absence of any affection at home. He is relieved to be able to confide in his physician and at this point decides to stop his weekly sexual flings when his son Francis comes home from college during the summer.

Rick finally chooses to leave Nicole. He asks her for a divorce, which catches her off-guard. Nicole never realizes why their marriage ends, or the part she may have played in its dissolution. On the outside, it seems so obvious both why Rick cheats and then insists upon a divorce. But while he is living his own story, he cannot see that the return of his sexual drive will ultimately be the undoing of his marriage. Nicole wants no part in their reunion as partners in any capacity. Rick has never considered this, and finds himself alone at the end, though happily content in the presence of his French bulldog.

Rick's pursuit of a better sex life is a solo endeavor. This is not uncommon in marriages where communication has eroded and sex becomes a distant memory. Often, one of the partners will insist on better sex, at the cost of finding it outside of the marriage. One could argue that Rick really tried to re-harness the spark within his marriage. He reached out to a sex therapist, but attended only three sessions, alone. One could also argue that Nicole's depression and entry into menopause were not legitimate reasons for Rick to have stepped out on their marriage. Both partners were having difficulties, but without any discussion as to why, they instead went on separate paths.

Rick's medical history of overcoming erectile dysfunction and the tale of his loveless marriage are the simplest of any of the characters. And yet Rick wrestles mightily with what to do at each turn. He is an example of how important sex is to humanity. Rick is not fulfilled with the sex he has with strangers. He finds it lonely to not have someone with whom to converse after coitus. He also despairs that his random sexual partners all have relationships they need to protect from discovering the motel room meetings, but he does not. Nicole is so disinterested in sex that she doesn't even have the energy to feel jealous anymore.

At the end of it all, Rick remains a likeable guy. His story represents millions of other marriages in mid-life, as he reports after his divorce when he goes out drinking with friends who are unhappy and are not having much sex either. Rick holds steady to what is important to him. If he can't have a good sexual relationship with a woman he can talk to, he would rather be alone. The addition of Rick finding a dog to ease the pain of his divorce was appropriated from a patient of mine who worked in the HVAC business. It was this guy who coined the phrase, *If you want sex, get a woman. If you want true love, get a dog.* Rick loves his French bulldog, and this pet seems to fulfill a lost sense of companionship. I have observed many men during hard times, and it seems that animals offer them a way to accept the nurturing they feel they cannot accept from other people. Perhaps more so than women, who have various relationships wherein they can feel weak and vulnerable, men respond to the presence of a pet by dropping their defenses and becoming softer and more loving by having a caring non-human sounding board for their weaknesses.

While it is a little sad that Rick winds up alone, he seems more content to be living without any expectation that his wife become someone that she is not. He also makes the honorable decision to leave a relationship that is unfair to everyone involved.

# Kirk

Kirk's character was loosely based on one of my patients who suffers from Chronic Pelvic Pain Syndrome. In keeping the identity of this patient safe, I will call him Sam. At the age of 25, Sam came to the pelvic floor physical therapy office with complaints of pain and burning along his urethra. His symptoms usually worsened with sex or prolonged sitting. Like Kirk, Sam desperately hoped that he had some sort of Sexually Transmitted Infection that could explain his symptoms. He was in a committed relationship then, and still is, so he worried about what the diagnosis of an STI would do to the fabric of his relationship. It turned out that Sam did not have an STI, which also filled him with grave concern about the nature of his penile pain.

After a few months of treatment in physical therapy, Sam almost fully recovered from his symptoms. He can now have pain-free sex and knows the triggers of his condition and what to avoid. In getting to know Sam, he admitted to me that he was on a swim team as a teenager in a local high school. The coach of the swim team was running an illegal and unethical underground business of selling Percocets to the team members. Sam began to buy these pills for musculoskeletal pain and very quickly found himself addicted. It wasn't until one day when the pills were no longer available (because the swim coach was fired and arrested), that one of Sam's friends went out and purchased a bag of heroin. Something inside Sam stopped him for joining that friend in getting high, and he has not touched opiates ever since.

One of Sam's greatest fears in learning about Chronic Pelvic Pain Syndrome, over a decade after his run-in with Percocet, was that he would be prescribed opiates and that the cycle of his addiction would return. Yet that never happened. Instead, Sam discovered physical therapy and was able to heal himself from his pelvic pain. It was during one evening in the clinic when Sam told me about his previous addiction when the character of Kirk seemed to materialize out of nowhere. Every time I treated my patient Sam thereafter, I would ask him what Kirk would do in any given situation. Should Kirk just use marijuana and booze for his pain, or should he descend into more addictive drugs? How would Kirk get off oxycodone once he had started? Finally, who would be the person to give Kirk enough hope to get clean?

Now, let's get back to the character Kirk. In the beginning of his story, we learn that he has no father figure in his life. The one thing that Kirk clings to from his Dad is his dream to become just like the drummer Don Henley from the band The Eagles. Kirk pursues this dream, though it becomes his undoing. His time on tour with the band coincides with the escalation of his pelvic pain. Kirk has no one he can talk to about his problem, he has no health insurance and cannot see a specialist and his addiction worsens in his feeble attempt to control the uncontrollable nature of his pain.

Kirk's inability to trust anyone was because of his father's departure in his young life. One of the reasons why the Eagles was chosen as the perfect band that Kirk tries to emulate is because they have a song about *everything*. (They really do.

They even have a song about a witch!) Their very poignant work, "Desperado", is one of the finest songs in this era of music which captures loss, addiction of any kind and the tendency of humanity to draw so far within ourselves that we cannot see anything but the terror of our own souls. Kirk's story is intertwined with this deep sense of isolation. He finds himself longing for his father on the long miles of the band's tour and plays this music to soothe what is forever gone.

Kirk's drug use only heightens this loss. But it is all that he believes he can do to heal the past and his own pelvic pain. The last straw is when Kirk snorts the crushed oxycodone pills in Alaska and blacks out during his evening with the Russian woman, Svetlana. The fear of the pain of having sex with her, coupled with the ending of the band's tour are what ultimately breaks Kirk down. It is then that Kirk hits his proverbial "rock bottom" and goes back to working at the gas station in New Jersey.

Kirk reunites with Ivan, the Russian Bear, who quickly realizes how far into trouble his young friend has gotten. Ivan gives Kirk his old job back, but he does something much more. Ivan gives Kirk a way to get off of opiates when he takes the young man to a doctor who prescribes suboxone. This is an excellent pharmaceutical which helps to ease the withdrawal symptoms of opiate addiction. Yet it is very expensive. Furthermore, many people in drug recovery can become addicted to suboxone as their new drug of choice. This is why the physician only prescribes Kirk two month's of suboxone and refuses any more. My patient Sam deserves sole credit for this turn in Kirk's story. "Very few people just choose to walk away from oxycodone. Kirk needs a way to find recovery, and suboxone is one way to do it," Sam advised. "Kirk also needs one person who believes in him. Someone to replace that piece of shit father who left him."

That was very the moment when Ivan, the Russian Bear, came into focus. We learn of Ivan's protective nature when Kirk remembers being a teenager and pumping gasoline. Ivan had gone to Kirk's high school graduation and stood in the bleachers with great pride. It is Ivan who saves Kirk at the end of the story as well. He invites Kirk over to his house on Saturday nights, and even refuses to drink vodka when his young friend comes over. That is a pretty big deal for a Russian who likes his drink. But that is how much Ivan loves Kirk. That is something a father would do for his son.

It is this connection between Kirk and Ivan that gives a measure of hope to an otherwise heartbreaking story. But this is what chronic pain can do to a person. It can lead to irrational thinking and cause terrible decisions to be made, out of desperation. When unmanaged, the path from pain to addiction is very short and dangerous. Through Kirk's story, however, we see that there is redemption and healing to be found, even in the darkest of circumstances. My patient Sam taught me that. Sam no longer needs physical therapy. But I thank him every time I think of him.

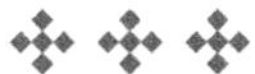

# Sheila

And now, without further ado, let's talk about everyone's favorite character, Dr. Sheila Ashtiju! The women with whom I work at the pelvic floor clinic refer to her as Sexy Sheila. Sheila is undeniably sexy, though that does not define her. What makes her such a fascinating woman is her keen intellect and her ability to make huge life changes that are aligned with her true nature.

The part of Sheila's story that marks her beginning is when she develops a friendship with Emily in high school. The two teenagers both adore science and chemistry lab. They study together and they don't compete with one another. Then one evening, Sheila and Emily have an unexpected dalliance into lesbian sex. It is after Sheila's discovery that she is attracted to Emily when she loses her friendship and must continue to hide who she really is.

When Sheila goes off to college and becomes a doctor, she dates men in order to appease her father. Farrouq is a traditional Muslim man who is very proud of his daughter. Well, he is very proud of who he believes is his *heterosexual* daughter. Sheila is once again torn between science (she is quickly rising to the zenith of her career as a urologist in Houston), and her sexual preference (she meets Stacy, the Operating Room nurse, and they pursue a full-on romance).

Sheila, clever as she is, decides to start her life over in a remote part of the country. Leaving her Muslim father allows her to relationship with Stacy to flourish in Pittsburgh. Because Sheila is so full of surprises, she also removes herself from her role as a surgeon and opens her own practice of treating men with sexual dysfunction. This is where we really get to see Sheila struggle with her life's decisions. On the one hand, she is thrilled to be in a place where she feels anonymous. On the other hand, Sheila grapples with her new line of work, the onset of her Seasonal Affective Disorder under the cloudy skies of Western Pennsylvania and her guilt about being a lesbian.

It was important that this book had the voice of a physician who treats one of the men. Through Sheila's eyes, we can see her unconventional methodology in helping men heal from their pelvic problems. As in many facets of her life, Sheila chooses to buck the system when it comes to her career. She removes herself from her status as a prominent surgeon and seeks a holistic approach to male sexual health. This is in keeping with Sheila's insistence that she can have a good life, on her own terms, without answering to anyone.

It isn't until Sheila's father Farrouq becomes ill that we see her fear in returning to Houston and facing her past. Sheila's girlfriend Stacy comes to the rescue and offers to drive Sheila down south. Stacy is self-aware enough to know that she won't meet Farrouq or attend his impending funeral. That is when the real shock happens. In his dying breath, Farrouq tells his daughter Sheila that he has always known that she was a lesbian. And that he loves her anyway.

Sheila is renewed by these words. They allow her to drive back to Pittsburgh and experience the magic of the Allegheny Mountains, to travel through the Fort Pitt Tunnel and to then emerge on the other side to see the glittering city that is now her home. Sheila also has a realization during that drive as to why she enjoys working with men. It is because she can see them as vulnerable humans, so vastly unlike her own father Farrouq. Yet even Farrouq becomes vulnerable at the end of his life, making jokes, eating pork products and accepting his daughter for who she is. Sheila is now set free from her past.

I know a physician who treats men for sexual dysfunction. The science behind how she does it is identical to Sheila's practice of medicine. It is this doctor who I channeled and bothered with countless questions, to help understand the role of hormones and the delicate blood chemistry required for male ejaculation. She is a very wise doctor and I commonly refer patients from the pelvic floor physical therapy clinic to go and see her. If Sheila is modeled after anyone, it is this brilliant physician, who also chooses to perform the art of medicine in her own way and refuses to be told what to do by a hospital system or insurance companies.

At the end of her story, Sheila's girlfriend Stacy suggests that they go to watch a Steelers football game. This is slightly ironic, as Stacy had been an ex-cheerleader for college football, and the Steelers have no cheerleaders. Yet Sheila becomes an unlikely fan of football, and this is in part because of the all-encompassing view she has of men. She can see them as tough and brutish while playing on Heinz Field, but she also knows that within each man is a teenaged boy, with fear and insecurity and the incredible pressure to be masculine and unyielding. To appear bigger and stronger than he really is.

When Dr. Sheila Ashtiju sees Rick for his final visit and her patient's erectile dysfunction is finally resolved, she tells him that she cannot continue to help him unless he allows himself to be happy. Rick takes this advice and divorces his wife. It is through the passing of her father that Sheila finally allows herself to be happy. I hope that the City of Pittsburgh considers the character of Sheila to be my formal apology for not recognizing its splendor from the very beginning.

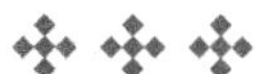

# Tom

I went to the Douro Valley in Portugal a few years back. This was before I specialized in the pelvic floor and I knew nothing about the delicate saddle muscles that control so many things for men. The Douro Valley is where the grapes are grown to make port wine. You haven't really seen Portugal until you've been to the Douro Valley. Traveling to the Iberian Peninsula and neglecting this gorgeous region is like going to the Empire State Building and not taking the elevator to the top floor.

While the views of the Douro River and Valley are stupendous and the farmers that live on these hills are industrious and welcoming people, it is the protection of the olive trees that stood out to me and begged to be written about. Remember that the grapes can be wiped out by the pesky insect known as Phyllox and this can destroy one season's worth of grapes in no time flat. It is the presence of an olive tree at the base of each row of grapes that can detect the nasty bug before it spreads throughout the fields. The olive tree is the Watchtower of the Grapes. This powerful metaphor was behind the creation of a character who was a sommelier.

Several years later, that character became Tom. Tom's story begins with a sudden onset of searing pain in his groin. He is successful and loves his job, he has a good marriage and two lovely daughters. But those things recede into the distance of his life and Tom's pelvic pain takes center stage. His life is consumed by it. He can no longer travel without pain, which is a large part of his job, his constipation is unrelenting, and the very thought of sex makes him hide away.

This is a classic representation of a patient with pelvic pain. The pain often begins suddenly and the symptoms "come out of nowhere". Many men find they cannot sit for any length of time, and in some cases, they last no longer than three minutes in a seated position before the pain surges and rectal spasms begin. A lot of patients report that their constipation is terrible and that they have severe pain after bowel movements. This leads to more constipation, as pain is now associated with going to the bathroom, so the brain unconsciously holds in stool to prevent further waves of discomfort. Lastly, a lot of men avoid sex once they have developed this level of discomfort. And just as Tom did, many of them don't tell their partners why they no longer want sex.

Unlike Kirk, who has no access to good healthcare, Tom does research and finds people who can help him with his pain. Dr. Nathan Shah is the first medical professional who Tom encounters that gets to the root of the problem. Tom then undergoes injections to his pelvic floor to decrease pain. Tom also finds a pelvic floor physical therapist named Sally. Both Dr. Shah and Sally play separate, yet integral and comingling roles in helping Tom address his problem.

Tom's psyche and mental state take quite a hit from his diagnosis of Chronic Pelvic Pain Syndrome. However, it is finally getting an accurate diagnosis that sets the ball rolling for Tom and gives him some hope. This is also very common in the real world of pelvic pain. Many men with these symptoms go to a variety of urologists and gastroenterologists looking for an answer, and none is given. It isn't until they get to the right

specialist and receive the correct diagnosis that they can begin the path towards healing.

There are doctors who perform the same injections to
the pelvic floor that Tom received from Dr. Nathan Shah.
Thankfully, these doctors have practices that are multiplying
and expanding, based on the diagnosis of pelvic pain becoming more mainstream and the information about this issue
more widespread. There are also an increasing number of pelvic floor physical therapists getting their requisite training to
help this ever-growing population of men who want to address
their problems.

Tom is a serious guy. While his job is that of a professional
wine-taster, which some people might perceive as a soft career
and not cut-throat or competitive, Tom has a Type A personal-
ity. This is characteristic of many men with pelvic floor tension;
they hold their body's anxiety in the small muscles of the saddle region. Everything Tom does in his life is precise and exact.
The way that he researches who to see for his pain and his
strict adherence to the instructions of his medical team reveal
a man who craves order and control. It is this same personal-
ity style that makes it such a challenge for Tom to ask for help
from his wife for his pelvic pain.

Tom eventually asks for help from his wife Casey. At the
end of his story, we learn that Casey has learned to do the rectal stretching that Tom receives in physical therapy, in order
to keep the pain from returning. While it is unusual to see this
happen in the real world of pelvic floor physical therapy, the
couples who are willing to do this are the ones with both the
strongest relationships and the best outcomes for managing
the pain. Pelvic floor PT's usually offer to train their patient's
partners to help improve the symptoms. Not a lot of men want

to place their partners in this position, which is unfortunate, because it would do wonders for their recovery, just as it did for Tom.

The character Sally is a nicely bubbled contrast to Tom's stern demeanor. As his physical therapist, she is enchanted by her job and her ability to help men in the most awkward of circumstances. Many pelvic floor physical therapists share Sally's enthusiasm for their trade and have undergone very undignified things to achieve their specialty (in order to learn about the rectum, pelvic floor PT's need to practice rectal stretching on each other). For this reason, they tend to be very open minded and able to talk freely about any topic, no matter how embarrassing. Sally is British in this story for one singular purpose: people from the U.K. refer to the rectum as the "back passage". It is such a wonderful turn of phrase, one that should be adopted in America, as "back passage" sounds so much better than rectum.

In the end, Tom learns to manage his pelvic pain. The culmination of his efforts is celebrated in the Douro Valley of Portugal, where he takes in the story of the olive trees as being the Watchtowers of the Grapes. It is here that he acknowledges the chronic nature of his pain. While it may never go away completely, Tom sees himself as a sturdy and loyal olive tree, waiting with vigilance to protect his body from the invasion of further pain. And because this analogy relates to wine, we see a more passionate side of Tom as lifts a glass of port in a toast to his great love Casey.

# Oliver

The character Oliver is a very interesting hybrid of masculinity. He is a mix of many things. For starters, Oliver is biracial. His father is a white American from the Deep South, while his mother is Jamaican. Oliver doesn't sense racism around him until his mother gets angry with his decision to join the Army. She fears that he is falling into a racial stereotype that minorities have no option other than the military. Yet Oliver very quickly rises in the ranks to being one of the best sharpshooters in his platoon.

Oliver takes great pride in his ability to handle firearms, all taught to him by his police officer father. It is in a field in Alabama when Oliver shoots the head off a turkey with precision at merely ten years of age. This is the beginning of his career as a marksman. Oliver looks back at that moment throughout his story and as he gets older and marries his wife Talulah, he often falls asleep while dreaming of shooting a gun. It's clear that Oliver is proud of his accomplishments and didn't even mind the hot desert of the Middle East in the earlier part of his journey.

Oliver's calm demeanor unravels very quickly with his diagnosis of prostate cancer. He hears the words of his doctor regarding the possibility of cancer, goes to his son's soccer game, and does not say one word. It is not until he arrives home to Talulah that Oliver becomes enraged and shouts from the shed in his backyard, while his wife attempts to protect their son from the kind of anger she has never yet witnessed in her husband. *"Fucking prostate cancer!? That asshole brought out the fucking battering ram, when it might not even BE cancer! He doesn't know what the fuck he is talking about! I don't have fucking cancer! How dare he say that to me!?"*

As a healthcare professional who treats many diagnoses, I have learned that there is something about the word cancer that changes people. Hearing the word cancer from a doctor's mouth is unlike getting any other news. I remember being a young physical therapist and I was required to treat patients in the hospital with various cancers. I was startled by their denial, their anger, and their anguish (and many of the patients were very close to my own age). I called my mother, who works as a Nurse Practitioner for patients with cancer. My mother is the type of person who "likes to throw cancer on the floor and stomp on it" (kind of like Dr. Sheila Ashtiju). I asked my mother why some people cannot not hear the word cancer without going into an existential tailspin, which often ends in a screaming match with their physicians.

"Oh, Becca," she replied. "Even the patients who don't scream at us when we tell them they have cancer are in complete denial. Everyone feels this way when they are first diagnosed. Some scream, others hide away and never come back for treatment, and some eventually take the treatment gracefully. But when a person first hears the word cancer, he or she thinks, *Other people get cancer. I don't have cancer. I simply don't.* Until they do have cancer. This is a very normal response. Because cancer can be such a mean-spirited disease, we as humans cannot believe that it has come for us."

It was because of my mother's wise words that Oliver's initial reaction to his cancer diagnosis was written as it was. After Oliver has the melt-down with his wife, he drives to his parents' house. Oliver sits in the backyard and drinks bourbon with his Dad, who has a history of being cured from prostate cancer and is doing okay. Oliver is itching to go out hunting to kill something, anything, but his father knows better than to allow this. Instead, Oliver and his father sit outside until the sun rises. Oliver then climbs into the bed of his childhood, while his mother cooks with intense worry about her son.

Once Oliver is officially diagnosed with cancer from a biopsy of his prostate, he registers this information as a man would. Slowly, in a measured pace, Oliver goes to his urologist and learns about treatment options. Like many men with prostate cancer, he wants to keep his prostate to maintain his sense of manhood. But just like many men with prostate cancer, he is fearful that cancer is growing in his body and wants to eradicate it with whatever treatment is most effective. Oliver chooses to have his prostate surgically removed. It is right before Oliver has surgery that he sees the faces of the Iraqi people as the targets at the end of his gun. Oliver is now stripped down to a very humble being.

He is reluctant to have sex after his surgery but is urged by his urologist to get back into the saddle. Oliver's wife Talulah is encouraging and in order to more fully understand what Oliver is going through, she joins a support group for partners of prostate cancer survivors. Oliver and Talulah adopt a son from Jamaica. This shift in the plot of Oliver's life is the sign of a survivor of cancer who realizes he will never sire any more children. It is the glimmer of acceptance. Oliver agrees to travel to an island and adopt another child who needs the security that he and his wife can provide. Another change within Oliver is his reluctance to shoot firearms. Due to his new and more mellow lifestyle, Oliver opts to use crossbows to teach his boys how to hunt. It is this gentleness within Oliver that reveals how his cancer has changed the way he lives and thinks.

This example of male "gentleness" is a very tricky line for men to navigate. Like Oliver, men have been historically expected to be aggressive protectors, hunters *par excellence*, financial providers, virile in the sack, and outwardly emotionally stoic, even in the wake of terrible news (like a cancer diagnosis). What we see in Oliver after his prostate is removed is someone who can be a generous and loving husband, a caring and attentive father and a man who accepts his fragility as a cancer survivor. Oliver's story begins with his image as being the stereotypical man. It ends with his new identity, a man who adapts to becoming a nurturer in addition to his role as protector.

In working with men who have been diagnosed with, are receiving treatment for, or are in the aftermath stage of prostate cancer, there are some specific qualities of this disease that are worthy of comment. First, when prostate cancer is detected early in its course, it is usually not a very fatal type of cancer. The survival rate for men who receive treatment for prostate cancer is very high. This should offer comfort to men diagnosed with it, but it often fails to do so, in the wake of the side-effects that often accompany the treatment of prostate cancer. Second, people are often in such a heightened state of panic when they receive a cancer diagnosis that they don't think about the side-effects of the treatment. Some patients are so intent on the destruction of the cancer cells within them that they don't ask enough questions or fail to get second opinions from other healthcare providers. Third, the patients who are aware of the side-effects of treatment, urinary incontinence and/or sexual dysfunction, don't feel comfortable talking about their diagnosis with friends or colleagues. This leads to a deep sense of isolation, which we can clearly feel from Oliver, even though Oliver has a supportive wife and parents. Lastly, many men with prostate cancer regain full recovery and have very few, if any, side-effects from the treatment. But the ones that do are plagued with a sense of failed manhood and virility. They say to themselves, *This cancer was supposed to be easy to beat. I am not going to die from this. But what will the rest of my life look like if I need to wear urinary pads or cannot have sex the way I used to?*

Oliver's character is meant to unveil the quandary that is prostate cancer. He is fortunate that his recovery is good, but he is still forever altered by his diagnosis. I wanted to give a voice to a man who embodies all of the salient qualities of his gender, yet who is forced to confront the loss of what he perceives to be the entirety of his masculinity. Rather than descending into this loss, Oliver comes to the realization that he is still very much a man after his surgery. Moreover, he is an even better provider and protector for those who he loves following his cancer. This is one of the greatest honors that I witness in my line of work. The Olivers that come through our doors are men who are afraid, shaken to their cores and completely vulnerable. After some time has elapsed and healing has occurred, these men emerge as true warriors. They are warriors who can still have sex, go back to work, and lead excellent lives. They are warriors who stare down the enemy of prostate cancer and society's expectation of themselves, eye to eye.

When I first started writing this book, my primary goal was to spread the knowledge about men with pelvic issues. But as I wrote and these characters developed their own identities, quirks, foibles and strengths, it occurred to me that I was writing to support all guys, whether they have pelvic problems or not. In today's world, there is a very high social cost to being a man. Men are expected to demonstrate their tough and strong qualities and to appear invulnerable. Men are often still expected to be primary financial providers in households. Men are tacitly disallowed from displaying tenderness and weakness, even though these qualities are precisely what women are longing to see within them. It is a confusing message, isn't it?

Remember the story in the introduction of this book about the cops of Newark, NJ? Everything about those men exemplified how we view men as a society. They wore dark blue uniforms with shiny badges and their weapons were strewn all over the office. Those men always knew where their own gun belts were located. They were protective of me, as their healthcare professional, and they were protective of each other. They were able to exchange information "on the sneak tip", the kind of private and covert intel regarding who was having an affair, who disliked working under a certain Captain in the department, and who was close to failing the semiannual firearm qualification. But none of them spoke of erectile dysfunction or testicular pain; definitely not urinary leakage or constipation. They would *never* discuss this with each other. That police department mirrored how men are supposed to act in the world. That is the image that they are held to, from young boys into adulthood. There existed no space for the police officers to talk about what was really going on in their lives. Unfortunately, this trend persists for men today.

Whenever I am treating male patients, I often ask them if they have confided in their families and partners about their pelvic problems. Many of them tell me no. It isn't because these men are insensitive. It is because they have been trained to be so strong and withholding that they cannot fathom talking about their weaknesses, especially when those weaknesses pertain to sex. The quote in the beginning of the third part of this book was from my friend, Henry Rolnik. "I'm not one for easy," he used to say. Henry was born in Poland before World War II, and as a Pole of Jewish ethnicity, he was the perfect target for the Nazi regime. Henry organized a small militia of fellow Polish men to fight and defend themselves and their families. Henry was captured with a fully loaded rifle by the Nazis and imprisoned in a Jewish work camp. Through a series of miracles and his own sheer will, Henry escaped from that prison camp and came to the United States by boat. He worked in the textile business, met and married his great love Katrina who died at 50 years of age from uterine cancer, and then retired to live with his grandchildren. I met Henry when he was 90. I learned of his life from his grandchildren, as Henry was not one to talk about what he had been through. Henry had lost most of his siblings during the war; they had died in Auschwitz. One would never know of Henry's difficult past from his broad smile and refusal to blame anyone for what had happened to him. The picture on the cover of this book is one of Henry's work boots. One can only imagine what ground those feet had covered. Henry was not one for easy. Neither are men with pelvic floor dysfunction.

The most crucial part of Henry's life story is how he formed that militia in Poland. While living in today's world, it is difficult to imagine Henry in the snowy mountains of Poland in the year

1939, banging on doors and convincing his fellow countrymen to leave their wives and children to fight against the Germans. But he did it. Henry must have been both persuasive and relentless as he went to each home. He never stopped fighting to defend himself and his land. Words were not what defined Henry; his action against what was wrong in the world did. I hope this book celebrates the kind of action that requires no description. I know the men that read this are leaving their comfort zones and banging on doors to protect themselves and the ones they love.

The challenge of being a man is today's world exists. To all the men out there, I hope you know that you are honored, in the way that you continue to fight without wavering, to struggle without complaining. I want to thank all the men who I have treated during my career. For your stories, your vulnerability, your trust. I especially want to thank those in law enforcement and the military; the reward for your efforts has not been fully expressed in recent times. This isn't an easy time to be a man. But you guys are not ones for easy. We need what you have to offer. Don't give up. Continue to protect us. Know that you are valued.

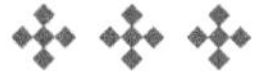

# Acknowledgements

A very special thank you to a certain American-Russian patient who I have been treating for chronic pelvic pain. He helped to guide me in writing about the "Soviet way". He also helped me to fully understand the pressures of a man with this kind of pain in the way that he supports his family without ever giving up.

Thank you to the dog who I got back in 2007. His name was Ruben and he had been a stud on a farm, impregnating the ladies with abandon, until I adopted him as a three-year-old. Ruben was my steadfast protector, just like the cops who surrounded me back then. He continued to protect me until he couldn't walk anymore. But we had a good twelve years together during which this creature showed me how incredible and necessary men are in the world.

A final thanks to the man who agreed to edit this book. Dave Bittner is the husband of my late sister Amy. Amy suffered from chronic pain during the end of her life. While it wasn't pelvic in nature, Dave and my family all bore witness to what pain can do to the mind and psyche of a person. Amy was wickedly smart and had wanted to edit one of my previous books, but she was too sick to be able to do it. When I called Dave early last winter and asked him to edit this book, he told me he had no experience with this type of job. I reminded Dave of what my sister Amy had told me about him. Dave could complete the Sunday *New York Times* crossword puzzle before Google was even a thing. That is how smart he is. I suppose that's why my sister married him. I thank Dave for continuing to be part of our lives with his wife gone. There is Amy in this book, for sure, and it was Dave who made certain of that.

# Bibliography

Allingham, C. (2017). *Prostate Recovery Map: Men's Action Plan 2*. Queensland, Australia: Redsok International.

Anderson, R. (2005). Integration of Myofascial Trigger Point Release and Paradoxical Relaxation Training Treatment of Chronic Pelvic Pain in Men. *The Journal of Urology*, 155-60.

Dorey, G. S. (2004). Randomized controlled trial of pelvic floor muscles and manometric biofeedback for erectile dysfunction. *British Journal of General Practice*, 54(508), 819-825.

Faubion, S. S. (2012). Recognition and management of non relaxing pelvic floor dysfunction. *Mayo Clinic Proceedings*, Vol 87, No. 2, pp.187-193. Elsevier.

Ferlay, J. H. (2010). Estimates of worldwide burden of cancer in 2008: GLOBOCAN 2008. *International Journal of Cancer*, 127, 2893-2917.

Frey, Glenn; Henley, Don. "Desperado". *Desperado*. Asylum, 1973. Record.

Goldstein, I. (2000). Male sexual circuitry. *Scientific American*, 283(2), 70-75.

Grunfeld, E. D.-C. (2013). "The only way I know how to live is to work": A qualitative study of work following treatment for prostate cancer. *Health Psychology*, 32(1), 75.

Kaplan, A. L., Hu, J. C., Morgentaler, A., Mulhall, J. P., Schulman, C. C., & Montorsi, F. (2016). Testosterone therapy in men with prostate cancer. *European urology*, 69 (5), 894-903.

Potts, J. (2003). Chronic Male Pain Syndrome: a nonpro statocentric perspective. *World Journal Of Urology*, 21 (2), 54-56.

Sathianathen, N. J., Johnson, L., Bolton, D., & Lawrentschuk, N. L. (2017). An objective measure of urinary continence with pelvic floor physiotherapy following robotic assisted radical prostatectomy. *Translational andrology and urology*, 6 (Suppl 2), S59.

Taylor, F. a. ( 2008). Non-surgical therapy of Peyronie's disease. *Asian Journal of Andology*, 10: 79-87.

Tries, J. &. (2005). The Use of Biofeedback for Pelvic Disorders Associated with a Failure to Relax. In M. S. Andrasik, *Biofeedback. A Practitioner's Guide* (p. 930). New York: The Guilford Press.

Van Kampen, M. D. (2000). Effect of pelvic floor reeducation on duration and degree of incontinence after radical prostatectomy: a randomised controlled trial. *The Lancet*, 355 (9198), 98-102.